# PATENTLY Erotic

# PATENTLY Erotic

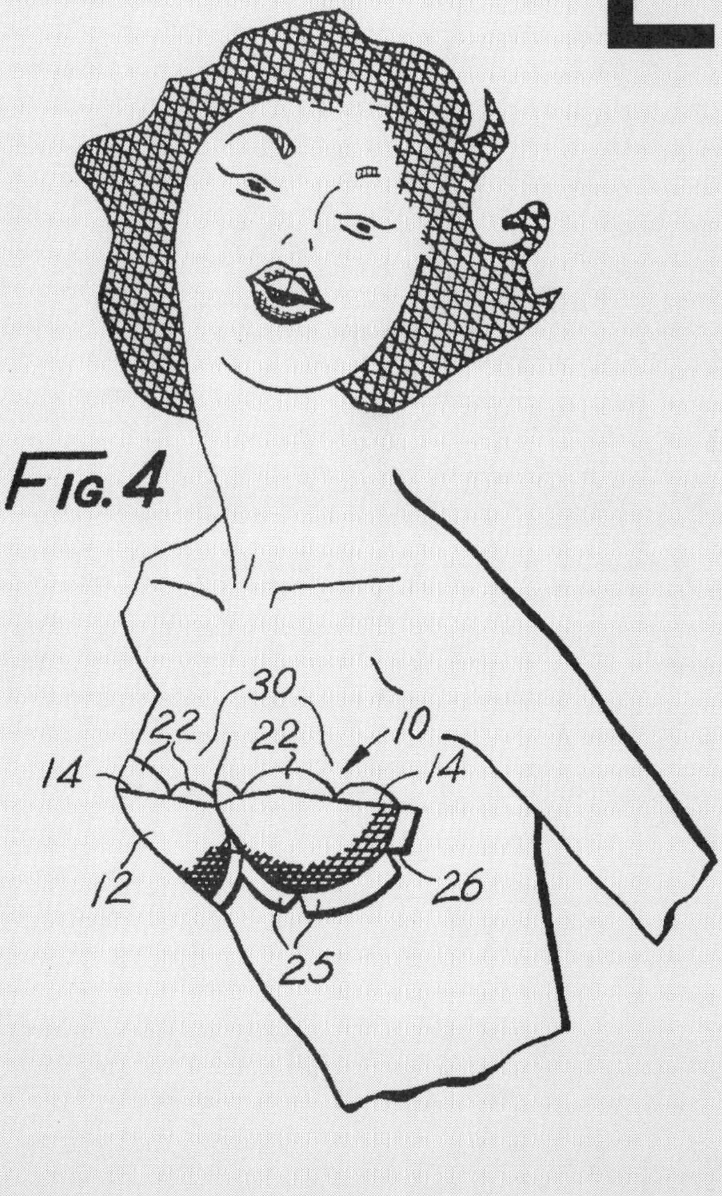

tear-away bras,
couple's chairs,
vibrating condoms
and other
patented strokes
of genius

**Richard Ross**

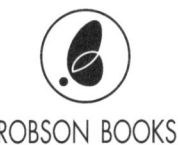

ROBSON BOOKS

This edition first published in Great Britain in 2005 by Robson Books, The Chrysalis Building, Bramley Road, London W10 6SP

An imprint of Chrysalis Books Group plc

First published in the United States by Plume, a member of Penguin Group (USA) Inc. in 2005.

Copyright © Richard Ross, 2005
Patently Erotic is a trademark of Richard Ross
The right of Richard Ross to be identified as the author of this work has been asserted by him in accordance with the Copyright, Designs and Patents Act 1998.

The author has made every reasonable effort to contact all copyright holders. Any errors that may have occurred are inadvertent and anyone who for any reason has not been contacted is invited to write to the publisher so that a full acknowledgement may be made in subsequent editions of this work.

British Library Cataloguing in Publication Data
A catalogue record for this title is available from the British Library.

ISBN 1 86105 910 8

All rights reserved. No part of this publication may be reproduced, stored in a retrieval system, or transmitted in any form or by any means, electronic, mechanical, photocopying, recording or otherwise, without prior permission in writing from the publisher.

Printed in Italy by Grafica Veneta S.p.A. - via Padova, 2 - Trebaseleghe (PD)
Original book design by Laura Lindgren

# contents

Foreword .................................. 8

Adhesive Brassiere and Its Method
    of Manufacture ...................... 10
Adult Sexual Apparatus ................. 12
Anal Orgasm Monitor .................... 14
Anatomical Device ....................... 15
Apparatus for Collecting Seminal Fluids ...... 16
Apparatus for Sexual Intercourse .......... 17
Article of Clothing for Use as a Condom ....... 18
Artificial Foreskin Device ............... 19
Artificial Vagina ........................ 20
Automated Masturbatory Device ........... 21
Auxiliary Erotic Implement ............... 22
Bedding with Multipe Overlays and Openings .. 23
Body Jewelry ............................. 24
Breast Protector ......................... 26
Breast Supporter ......................... 27
Chair Device for Enhancing Sexual Intimacy ... 28
Coitus Assistance Device for Males ......... 30
Condom ................................... 31
Condom for Oral-Genital Use .............. 32
Condom with Multi-Purpose Sexual Device ... 34
Condom with Spiral Crisscross Ribbing ...... 35

Conductive Condom ....................... 36
Couple's Chair ........................... 37
Decorative Penile Wrap ................... 38
Device for Assisting and Maintaining
    an Erection ......................... 40
Device for Use in Human Copulation ........ 41
Device to Enhance Clitoral Stimulation
    During Intravaginal Intercourse .......... 42
Disposable Tear-Away Brassiere ........... 43
Ear Fastener for Oral Condoms ............ 44
Electrical Appliance for Assisting Anatomical
    Organs .............................. 45
Electromechanical Massager Apparatus ...... 46
Erection Holder .......................... 47
Erogenic Stimulator ...................... 48
Erotic Stimulation Device (Tongue Roller) ..... 49
Erotic Stimulator ........................ 50
External Device for Eluding Masculine
    Impotence ........................... 51
External Penile Prosthetic Device ......... 52
External Vibratory Exercising Device for
    Pelvic Muscles ...................... 54

| | |
|---|---|
| Female Condom . . . . . . . . . . . . . . . . . . . . . . . . | 55 |
| Female Garment . . . . . . . . . . . . . . . . . . . . . . . | 56 |
| Female Stimulator Comprising Close-Fitting Clitoral Suction Chamber. . . . . . . . . . . . . . | 58 |
| Feminine Napkin Allows External Sexual Intercourse. . . . . . . . . . . . . . . . . . . . . . . . . | 59 |
| Glandular Stimulator Device and Method. . . . . . | 60 |
| Hair Circle for Conjugal Affection. . . . . . . . . . . . | 62 |
| Hydro-Therapeutic Stimulator . . . . . . . . . . . . . | 63 |
| Improvement in Uterine Supporters . . . . . . . . . | 64 |
| Intercourse-Facilitating Therapeutic Furniture . . | 65 |
| Kissing Shield and Method of Use Thereof. . . . . | 66 |
| Lap Dance Liner. . . . . . . . . . . . . . . . . . . . . . . . | 68 |
| Lingual Vibration Device . . . . . . . . . . . . . . . . . | 69 |
| Lover's Game and Method of Play . . . . . . . . . . | 70 |
| Male Garment with Scrotal Pouch . . . . . . . . . . | 72 |
| Male Genital Device and Method for Control of Ejaculation . . . . . . . . . . . . . . . . . . . . . . | 73 |
| Male Genital Strengthening Device . . . . . . . . . | 74 |
| Male Organ Conditioner . . . . . . . . . . . . . . . . . | 75 |
| Male Organ Jacket . . . . . . . . . . . . . . . . . . . . . | 76 |
| Male Sexual Aid Holder. . . . . . . . . . . . . . . . . . | 77 |
| Massage Apparatus . . . . . . . . . . . . . . . . . . . . | 78 |
| Massage Device . . . . . . . . . . . . . . . . . . . . . . . | 80 |
| Massaging Apparatus for Penis. . . . . . . . . . . . . | 82 |
| Massaging Apparatus (with Stroking Device) . . . | 83 |
| Men's Anatomic Underwear/Swimwear. . . . . . . | 84 |
| Method for Decorating a Human Breast. . . . . . . | 86 |
| Method of Inducing Safety in Sexual Acts and Aids in Support Thereof. . . . . . . . . . . . . . . | 88 |
| Method of Sexual Disharmony Correction During the Sexual Act . . . . . . . . . . . . . . . . | 89 |
| Mood Lamp . . . . . . . . . . . . . . . . . . . . . . . . . . | 90 |
| Multifacet Sexual Aid . . . . . . . . . . . . . . . . . . . | 91 |
| Nipple Pad . . . . . . . . . . . . . . . . . . . . . . . . . . . | 92 |
| Oral Prophylactics . . . . . . . . . . . . . . . . . . . . . | 94 |
| Panty Condom . . . . . . . . . . . . . . . . . . . . . . . . | 96 |
| Penile Erection Aid . . . . . . . . . . . . . . . . . . . . . | 98 |
| Penile Prosthetic Apparatus . . . . . . . . . . . . . . | 100 |
| Penis Surgical Splint. . . . . . . . . . . . . . . . . . . . | 102 |
| Plug and Phallic Device and System . . . . . . . . . | 103 |
| Portable Vibrator . . . . . . . . . . . . . . . . . . . . . . | 104 |
| Prophylactic Device (Condom). . . . . . . . . . . . . | 105 |
| Prophylactic Device (Underwear). . . . . . . . . . . | 106 |
| Prostate Gland Massaging Implement. . . . . . . . | 108 |
| Prosthetic Appliance. . . . . . . . . . . . . . . . . . . . | 109 |
| Protective Mask . . . . . . . . . . . . . . . . . . . . . . . | 110 |
| Reinforced Tethered Condom Construction. . . . . | 111 |
| Rolling Ring Condom . . . . . . . . . . . . . . . . . . . | 112 |
| Self-Contained Gynecologic Stimulator . . . . . . . | 113 |
| Sensory Transmitting Membrane Device . . . . . . | 114 |
| Sex Aid . . . . . . . . . . . . . . . . . . . . . . . . . . . . . | 115 |
| Sex Aid Device for Males. . . . . . . . . . . . . . . . . | 116 |
| Sex Couch . . . . . . . . . . . . . . . . . . . . . . . . . . . | 117 |
| Sexual Aid . . . . . . . . . . . . . . . . . . . . . . . . . . . | 118 |
| Sexual Aid Device . . . . . . . . . . . . . . . . . . . . . . | 120 |
| Sexual Aid (Strap-On). . . . . . . . . . . . . . . . . . . | 121 |
| Sexual Appliance Having a Suction Device Which Provides Stimulation. . . . . . . . . . . . . | 122 |
| Sexual Device for Handicapped Men . . . . . . . . | 123 |
| Sexual Erection Prosthesis and Method of Use. . . . . . . . . . . . . . . . . . . . . . . . . . . . | 124 |
| Sexual Stimulation Apparatus. . . . . . . . . . . . . . | 126 |
| Sexual Stimulator. . . . . . . . . . . . . . . . . . . . . . | 127 |

| | |
|---|---|
| Spreader Means Garment.................. 128 | Therapeutic Aid Apparatus and Method....... 136 |
| Stimulator .......................... 130 | Therapeutic Brassiere..................... 137 |
| Strap On Condom...................... 131 | Thrusting Rod......................... 138 |
| Strap Secured Condom.................. 132 | Vacuum Driven Stimulative Sexual Aid ....... 140 |
| Surgical Applicance .................... 133 | Vaginal Shield for Preventing Sexually |
| Swinging and/or Spinning, Hanging Seat for | Transmitted Diseases ................ 141 |
| Erotic Purposes .................... 134 | Vibrating Condom....................... 142 |
| Therapeutic Adapter ................... 135 | Vibrator System ....................... 143 |

# foreword

> "If you build it, he will come."
> Ray Kinsella, *Field of Dreams*

REMOTE CONTROLLED VIBRATING UNDERPANTS. Four simple words. Strung together, they suggest not only a wonderfully strange product, but an unusual mind behind that product. Say the words gently: they roll off the tongue, filling one's mind with delicious visions.

Remote controlled vibrating underpants. Someone, somewhere, thought this was a really, really good idea. Such a good idea, in fact, that the inventor filed paperwork, paid a substantial fee, and registered his or her idea for eternity, protecting it from those who might attempt to copy it. And so, somewhere in the depths of the U.S. Patent Registry, is Patent Number US 6,553,266 B1, for underpants that allow one to stimulate a woman from across the room with a remote control.

Patent applications are filed by people of all countries, citizens of all states. Inventors are male and female, all ethnicities, all ages. But what kind of person imagined such a wondrous device as vibrating underpants? Who believed there might be a commercial demand for such a product, justifying the spending of real money to register its patent?

Most important, where can I buy a pair?

There is little as simple—or as complicated—as sex. Functionally, it is your basic Tab A into Slot A. But this hasn't stopped man (and woman) from attempting to build a better mousetrap. While dildos have existed for thousands of years—used mainly for ritual and ceremony—the technological revolution of the twentieth century gave men and women the previously unknown treasure of free time. With free time comes time to imagine, and when men and women have time to imagine, it's inevitable someone will come up with the talking condom.

India has a history of sexual exploration. The *Kama Sutra* offers directions on the many facets of sexual embrace where the sexual and the sacred together are the weaver of the tapestry of life. Positions include: Mare's Position, Suspended Congress, The Somersault, The Ostrich's Tail, Drawing the Bow, Camel's Hump, Blacksmith's Posture, Dragon Turns Over, The Phoenix Flutters, Cranes with Necks Intertwined, and many others. The inventiveness has the innocence and sophistication of being organic. They look to the body itself and the permutations that can occur within the sphere of the flesh. Inventiveness is not a uniquely western nor eastern phenomena. But it is notable that while India looked to the natural world for diversity of coupling, the West began its investigation with the "D" cell battery.

The first U.S. patent was issued on July 31, 1790, for a soapmaking technique. It was not sex-related, except inasmuch as the end product of soapmaking tends to increase one's likelihood of scoring. But it wasn't long before steam power, conveyor belts, and automatic pulleys began to be assembled for the purpose of hitting those...hard-to-reach areas. The portable massager of the early twentieth century, for example, seemed suspiciously rigorous in its instructions—so rigorous, in fact, that the back-and-forth motion of the massaging piston demanded the apparatus be anchored to a table.

More dynamic changes have occurred as miniaturization and battery-powered instruments became more common. Just as the radio shrunk from furniture to hand-held device, so too did the sex toy. The liberation of the 1960s meant that sex was celebrated with all its bells and whistles—literally, in the case of some of the era's patents. Tab A and Slot A were just the beginning: there was an alphabet's worth of tabs and slots out there, and each one had an entrepreneur building the perfect pleasure device for it.

Vibrators are now handheld, with physical appendages designed by women to respect the architecture of their anatomy. And once you've invented that, why not add lights to enhance the mood? And once you've added lights, why not sound systems, to play the sound of a lover's voice (or, as preferred by most users, the voice of Al Green)?

Even as we rocket into the twenty-first century, however, some inventors still prefer to keep it simple. Electronic devices have no place in the world of the uni- or bi-sexual leather harness apparatus. And sometimes the most charming inventions are the most basic: witness the wrap that sheaths the penis in the guise of Frosty the Snowman or (for those not in the festive spirit) the grim reaper.

Every day, patent applications are filed to protect the creativity of individuals describing human genome sequences as well as chastity belts; technologies to enhance weaponry or space travel as well as mechanical penis chin straps. The patent office is a depository that documents the places where "no man has gone before."

This book is a testament to the bored woman sitting on a washing machine with an energetic spin cycle; to the construction worker with a jackhammer and an overactive imagination. This book is a celebration of innovation at its most feverish, a loving catalog of a century's worth of wondrous strokes of genius.

# Adhesive Brassiere and Its Method of Manufacture

Patent No. 4,343,313
Aug 10, 1982
Danielle Le Jeune

### Abstract

The brassiere is composed of two symmetrical elements, each supporting one breast. The element comprises a wide part adhesively positioned under the breast and/or on the side, and a thin shoulder-strap adhering, at least at the end, to the back part of the shoulder. The brassiere may be attached to clothing, if desired, to support the same.

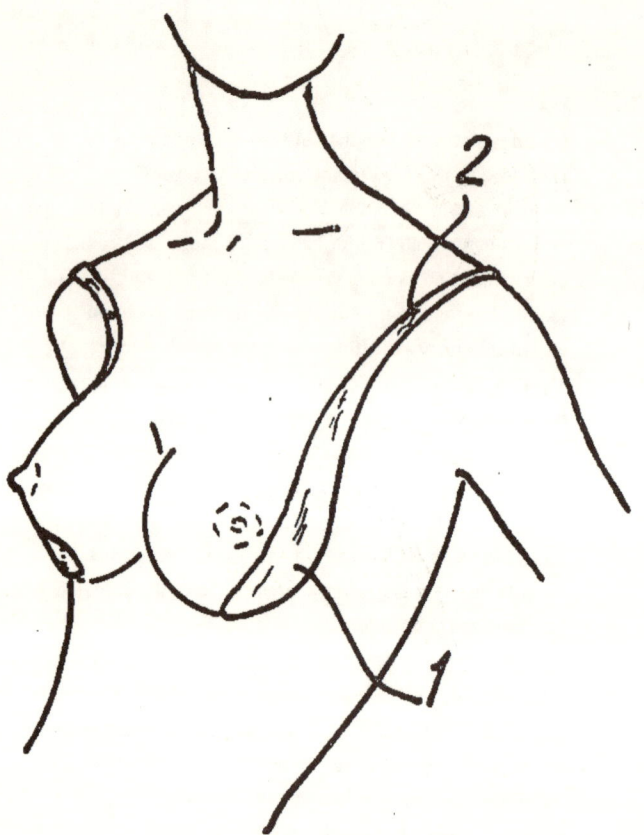
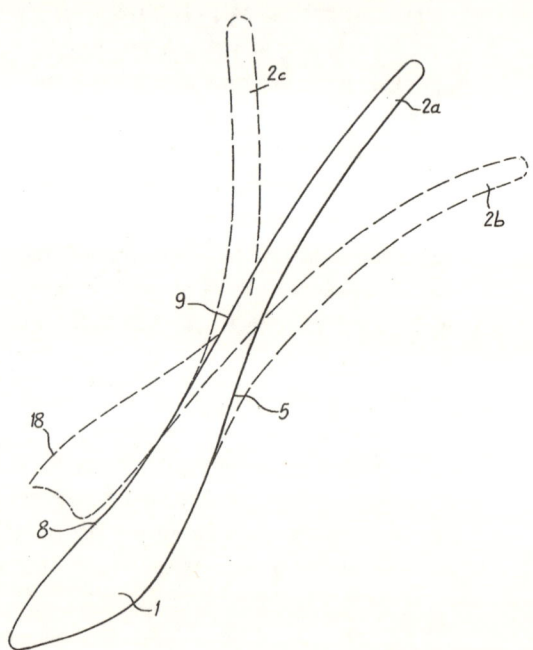

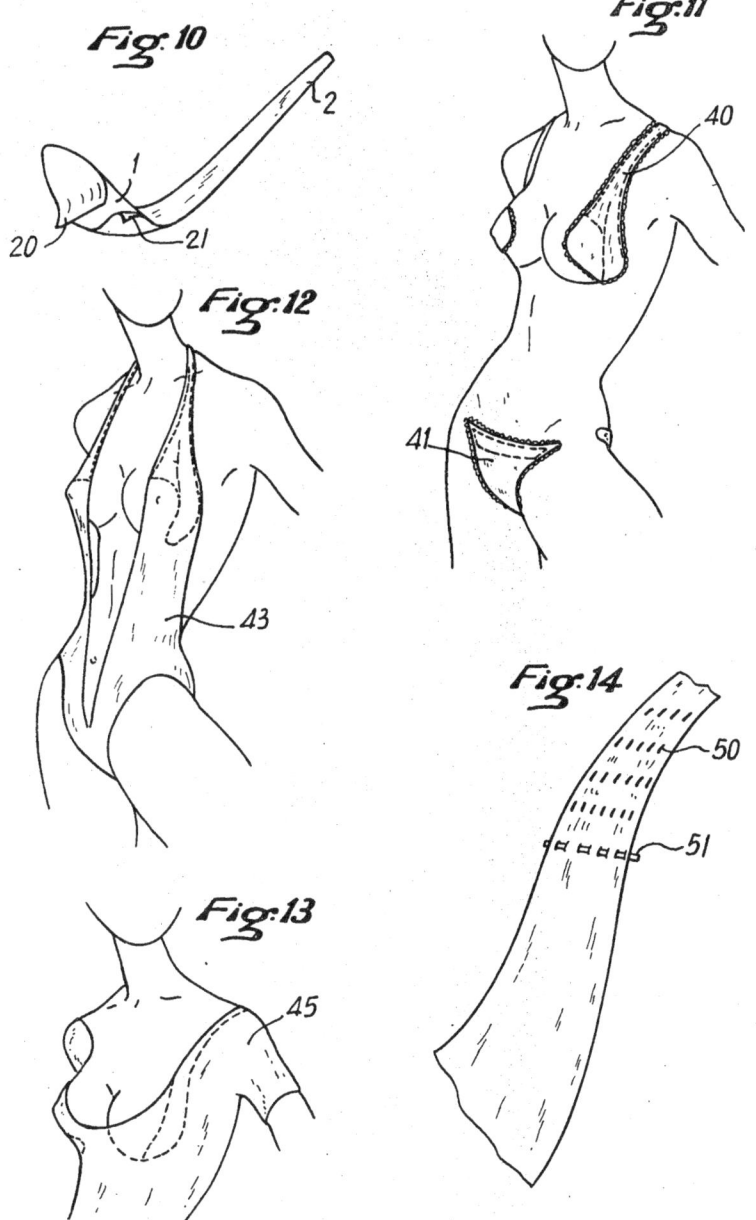

Patent No. US 6,203,491 B1
Mar 20, 2001
Richard M. Uribe

# Adult Sexual Apparatus

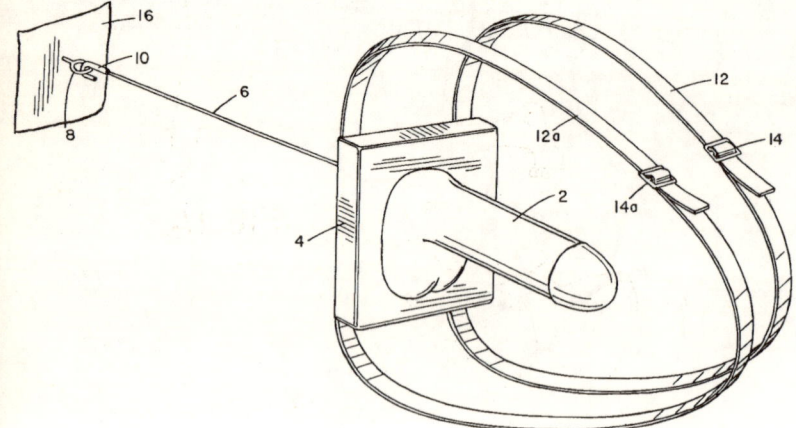

## Abstract

An improved hands-free adult sexual apparatus or adult toy for use by women or men. The apparatus is secured onto the user, or the user's clothing or belt, in a harness-like assembly and is also partially restrained to a fixed object. In one embodiment, a dildo or other phallic device is secured to a supportive backing while elastic straps allow the user to comfortably utilize the invention. A restraining line partially secures movement of the dildo or phallic device while the user manipulates the elastic straps. In another embodiment, the phallic device has a lubricant chamber that is activated by a user controlled trigger to permit the user to add lubricant as desired to the phallic device. In another embodiment, the invention has instead a sheathing device for use by males.

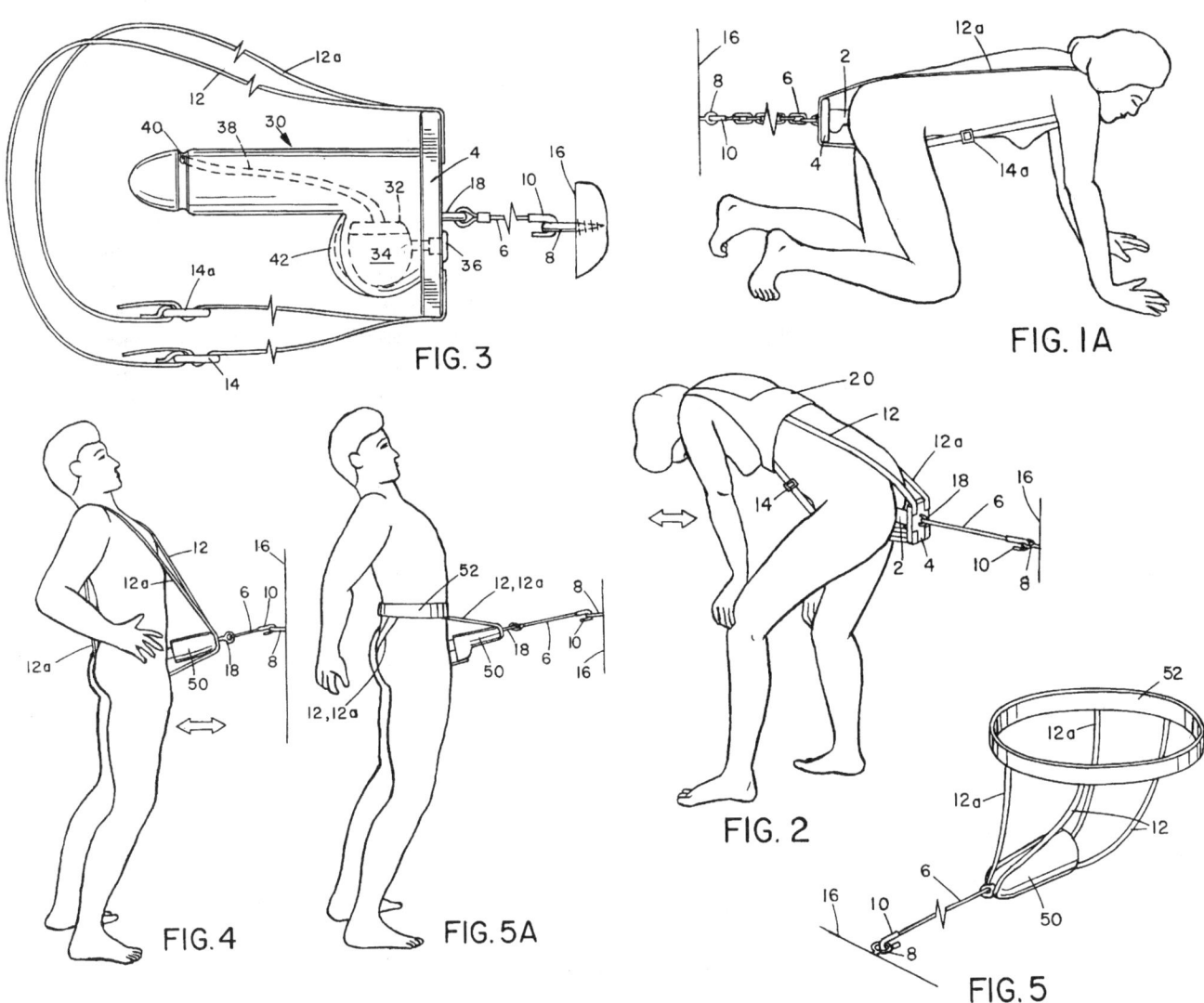

Patent No. 5,787,892
Aug 4, 1998
James Conway Dabney

# Anal Orgasm Monitor

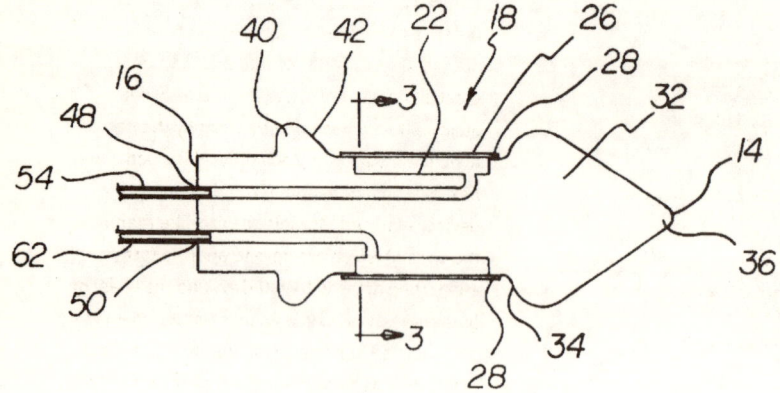

## Abstract

A device for determining the contractions of an anal sphincter and associated muscles comprising a core formed in a generally cylindrical configuration from a relatively rigid plastic material having a distal end and a proximal end, the core having a central section of a reduced diameter and an axial length, sheet material formed of a flexible essentially inelastic plastic material with an adhesive securing the sheet material to the core and a head adjacent to the distal end of the core, the proximal end of the head being located adjacent to the distal end of the central section and with the distal end of the head being of a reduced diameter.

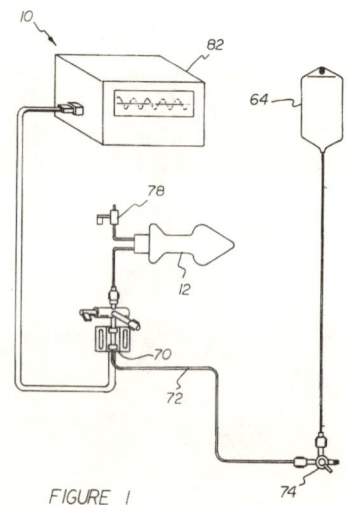

FIGURE 1

Patent No. 4,440,183
Apr 3, 1984
Jess Miller

# Anatomical Device

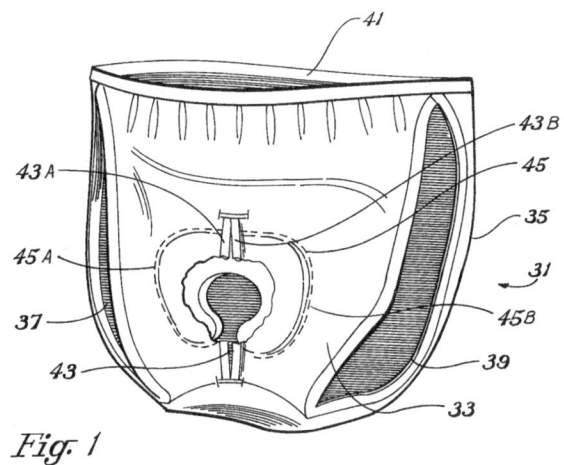

Fig. 1

## Abstract

A device to be fitted around the penis of a human male to facilitate and maintain an erection. In one embodiment, the device is attached to a garment to be worn by the person to hold the device in place around the penis and next to the body. In another embodiment, the device is formed by a folded wire-like member the ends of which are spread apart to form supporting arms to be fitted around the waist or hips of the person. In a further embodiment, a belt, adapted to be secured around one's waist, is attached to the wire-like member for holding it in place.

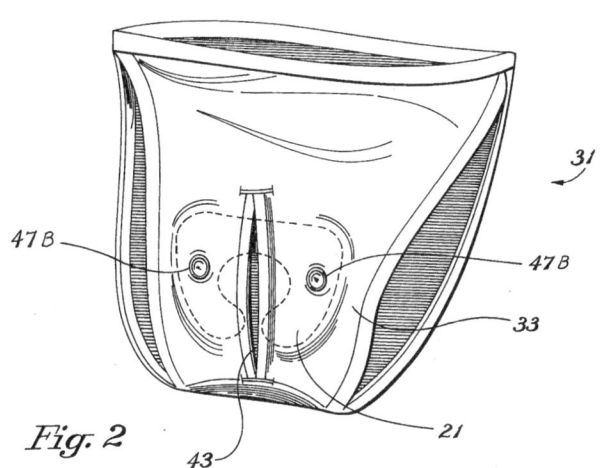

Fig. 2

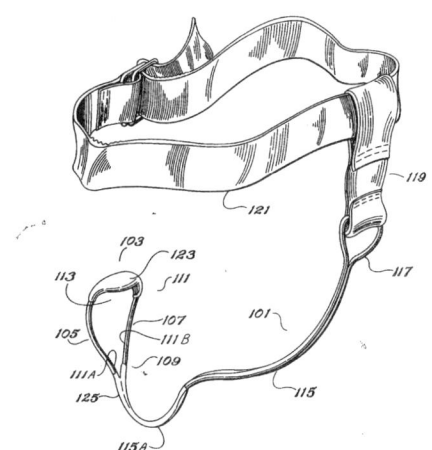

Patent No. 4,312,350
Jan 26, 1982
Rosetta C. Doan

# Apparatus for Collecting Seminal Fluids

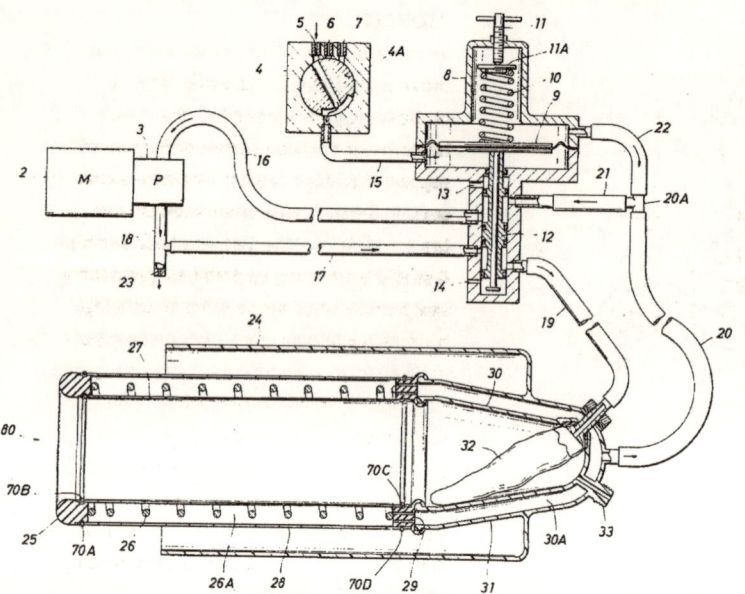

## Abstract

Method and apparatus for collecting seminal fluid for artificial insemination is provided and wherein the apparatus has a flexible wall closed at one end and with a rim at the other open end movable in a reciprocating fashion back and forth with respect to the closed end wall. An inflatable sphincter member is located within the vagina adjacent the closed end and applies pressure to the penis during thrusting actions by the animal.

Patent No. US 6,640,808 B1
Nov 4, 2003
Jeffrey E. Fessler

# Apparatus for Sexual Intercourse

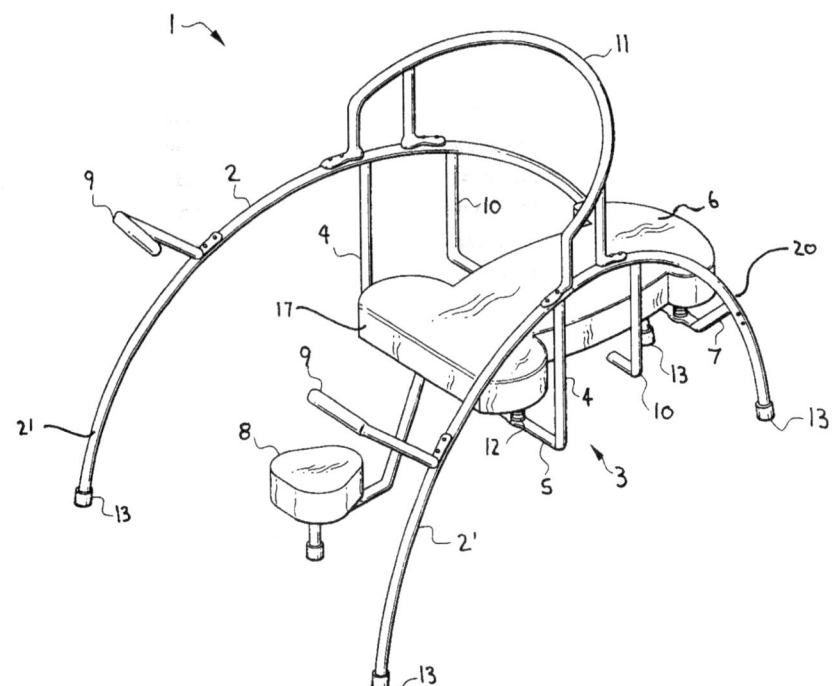

## Abstract

An apparatus for sexual intercourse includes two arcuate-shaped legs connected by a centrally located brace and another brace located near the head portion of the padded support. A padded support for a non-dominant sexual partner is located between the two braces, to support the partner's head and hips. A seat is located for the dominant partner, the seat being located between the arcuate legs near the hip portion of the flat padded support. A handrail is located above the flat padded support such that it is within easy reach of either participant. Supine footrests are located in front of the hip portion of the padded support for use when the non-dominate partner is in a supine position. Upright footrests are also located near the center of the flat padded support for use in other sexual positions.

# Article of Clothing for Use as a Condom

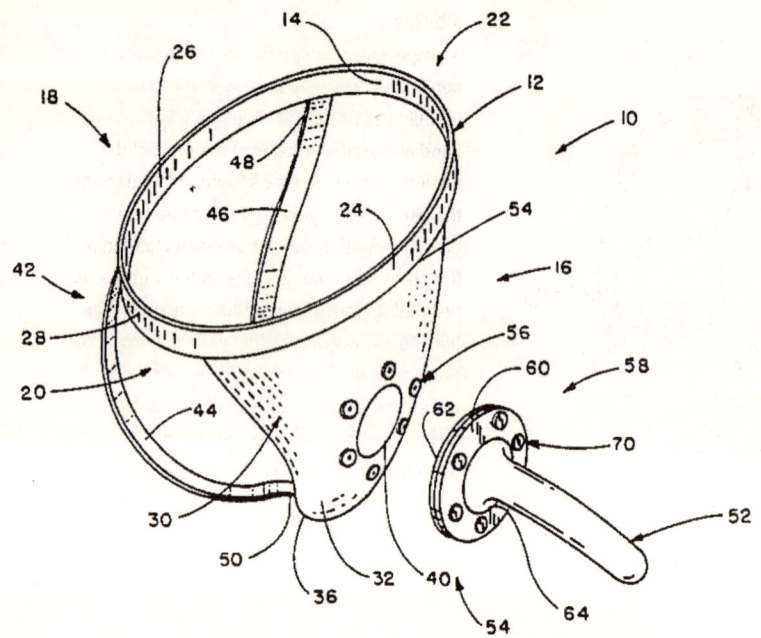

Patent No. 4,942,885
July 24, 1990
Anton Davis; Kelvin A. Simmons; Richard Blair

### Abstract

An article of clothing prevents transmission of sexually-transmitted diseases, such as infestation of Phthirius Inguinalis to the pubic area of the wearer. The article of clothing includes a codpiece-like element that has snaps thereon for releasably attaching a condom mounting plate assembly to the codpiece-like element. A condom is held in the plate assembly.

Patent No. 5,074,315
Dec 24, 1991
James J. McCuiston

## Artificial Foreskin Device

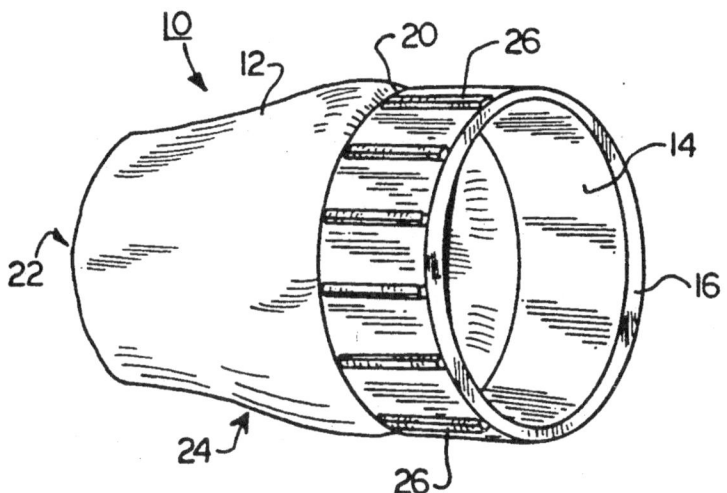

### Abstract

A prophylactic device adapted to be worn on a penis. The device includes a bottle-shaped, tubular sheath open at both ends and an elastic band attached along one of the ends of the sheath for securing the sheath to the glans of the penis. The tubular sheath is operable to prevent constant contact between clothing and the glans of the penis while, at the same time, permitting normal micturition functions. The band is relatively thick and wide to form a roll-preventing perimeter and further includes raised, generally longitudinally extending ribs arranged about the outer surface of the band for preventing the band from rolling up.

Patent No. 5,458,559
Oct 17, 1995
Arthur E. Gauntlett

# Artificial Vagina

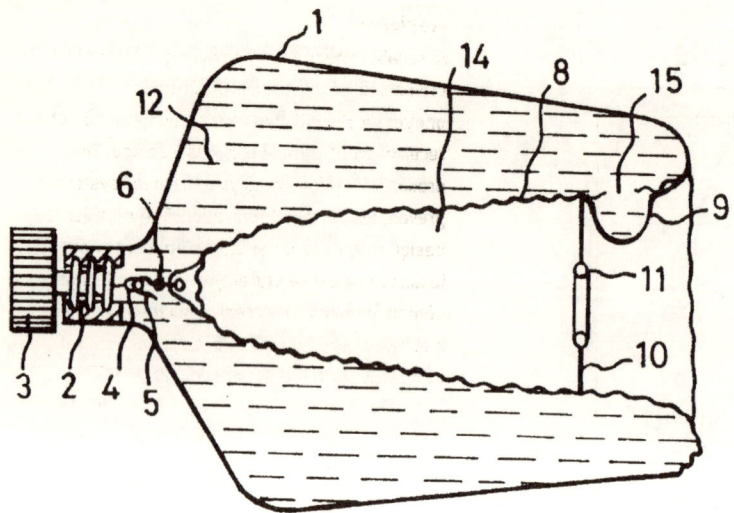

## Abstract
An artificial vagina is described includes a sheath made from a flexible waterproof material. The sheath tapers from one end to the other, the wider end having a releasable opening closed by a screw-threaded stopper. Projecting from the inner end of stopper is an eye loop connected to a hook which swivels on wire loop secured to tab. The tapered end of sheath has a soft flexible undulating wall and a bulbous portion from which extends an annular membrane, the peripheral edge of which has a reinforced elastic rib. When assembled with the hook connected to wire loop a fluid chamber is formed and filled with warm water forming a chamber. Aperture is formed in wall to connect with bulbous portion for the passage of the water.

Patent No. 5,501,650
Mar 26, 1996
Reinhard R. Gellert

## Automated Masturbatory Device

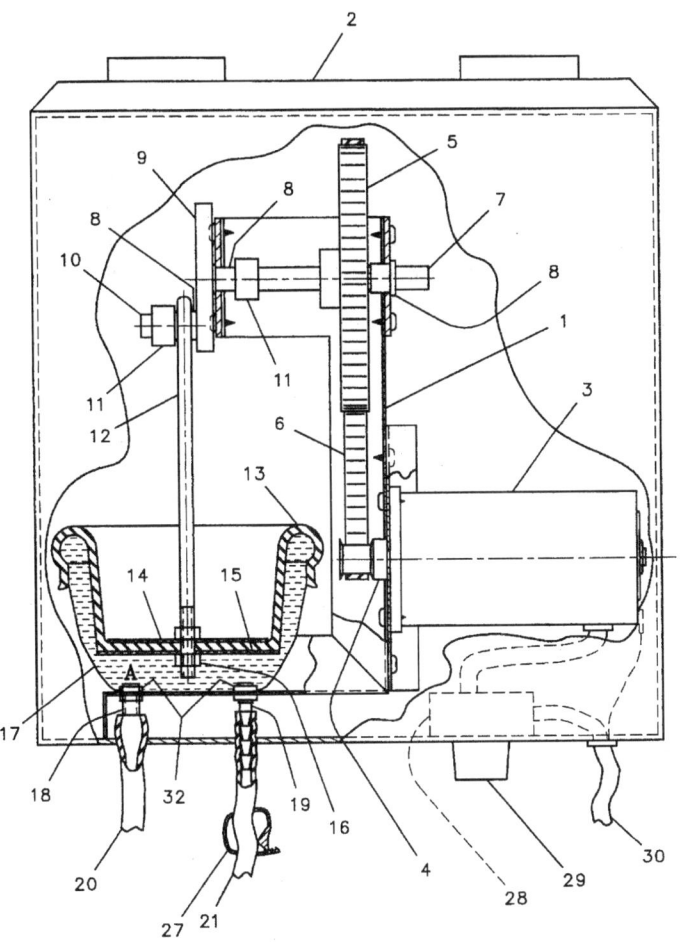

### Abstract

A variable speed motor powering a crankshaft driven sealed transducer producing pneumatically induced reciprocating motion of a receiver when a male organ is inserted. The present invention employs a hermetic system to prevent loss of synchronization. The receiver is designed with an inner liner compliant enough to accommodate a plurality of sizes and shapes of male penises. The present invention produces a stroke of approximately 3 inches at a frequency of up to 350 per minute.

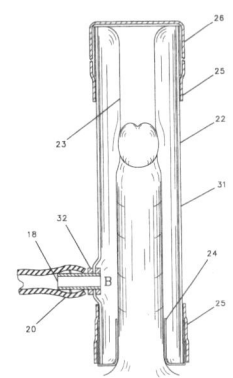

FIG. 3a

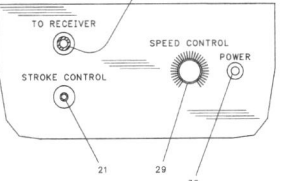

Patent No. US 6,190,307 B1
Feb 20, 2001
Chi-Wen Tsai

# Auxiliary Erotic Implement

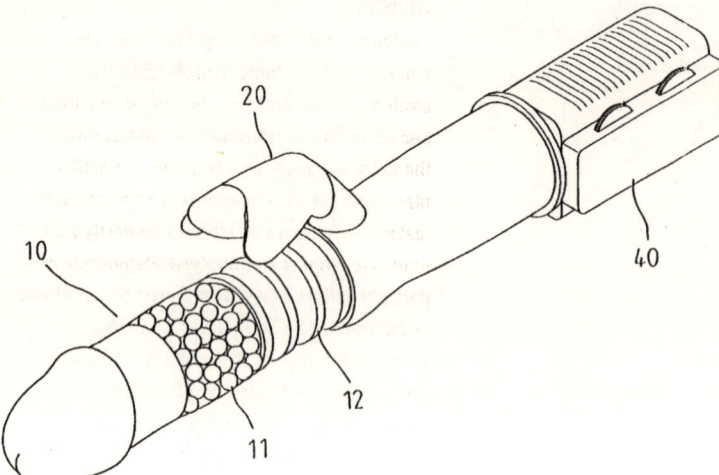

## Abstract

An auxiliary erotic implement includes a body, a vibrator, a transmitting unit, and an changeover switch. The body has an intermediate portion provided with a layer of rolling beads under the surface, and the vibrator provided on an outer surface of a rear portion. The transmitting unit is contained in the body, consisting of a motor, tow gear and rod sets, a slide plate, an interacting gear and an interacting rod. The body is rotated for 360° and moves axially back and forth at the same time by the two gear and rod sets rotated by the motor controlled by the changeover switch and cooperated by the interacting gear, the interacting rod and the slide plate. In addition, the rolling beads also roll together with the body, enhancing worth of the implement and pleasure to be acquired.

Patent No. US 6,640,362 B1
Nov 4, 2003
Carlton H. Kimball

# Bedding with Multiple Overlays and Openings

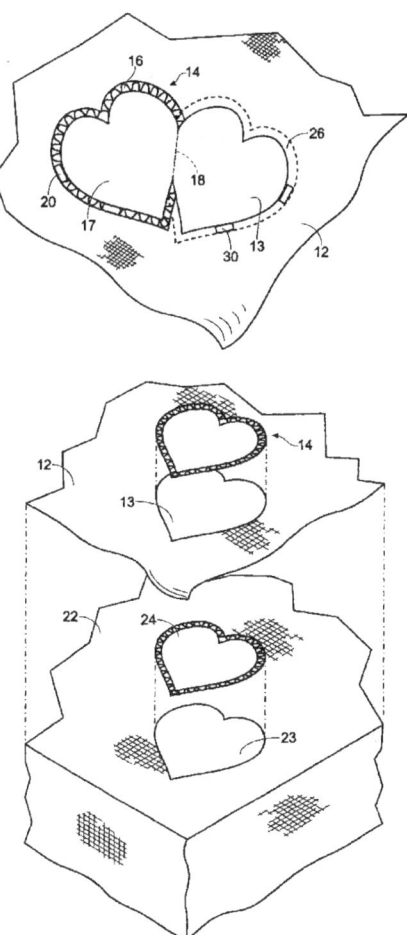

## Abstract

Complimentary articles of bedding with cut-outs and removable or hinged opening overlays strategically located over the erogenous areas of bed occupants for purposes of enhancement of the sensual experience. Overlays are held in place over cut-outs or exposure openings with fasteners. Overlays attached to, or partly cloth hinged to blanket and/or sheet. Removable or partially openable at will by one or both partners as activities of an amorous nature may progress. Progressively smaller openings and overlays from top to bottom for a series of coaxially aligned openings and overlays in a mated sequence of bedding materials.

Patent No. 5,784,900
July 28, 1998
Patrick Czupryniak

# Body Jewelry

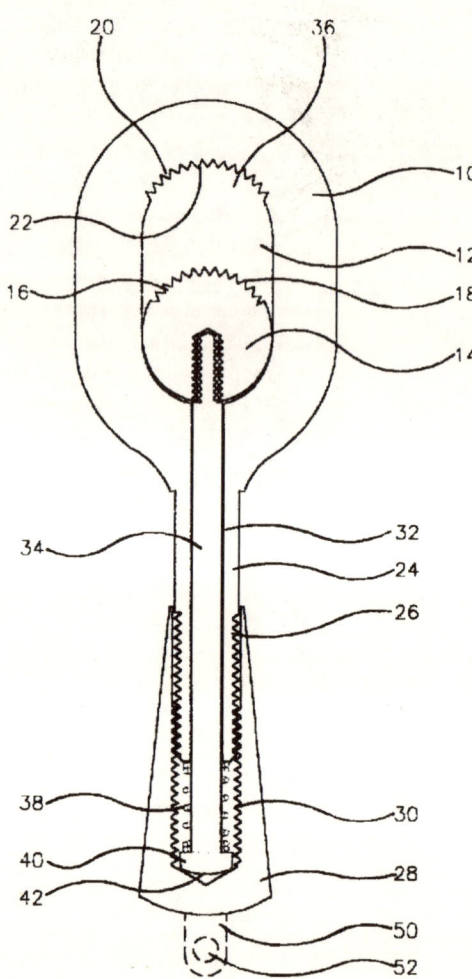

## Abstract

A jewelry device comprises a unitary body having defined therein an aperture, a clamping member disposed within the aperture, and a shaft for displacing the clamping member between an open position and a closed position within the aperture. The aperture is sized to accommodate a part of the body to be decorated, such as the nipple of a breast, when the clamping member is in the open position. Once a nipple has been inserted into the aperture, the shaft is displaced so as to bring the clamping member into contact with the nipple, and thus grip the nipple. The device allows the strength of the grip exerted on the nipple to be varied. The device may be plated with a precious metal, and may be provided with any combination of adornments such as jewels, spikes, and studs, to increase its aesthetic appeal.

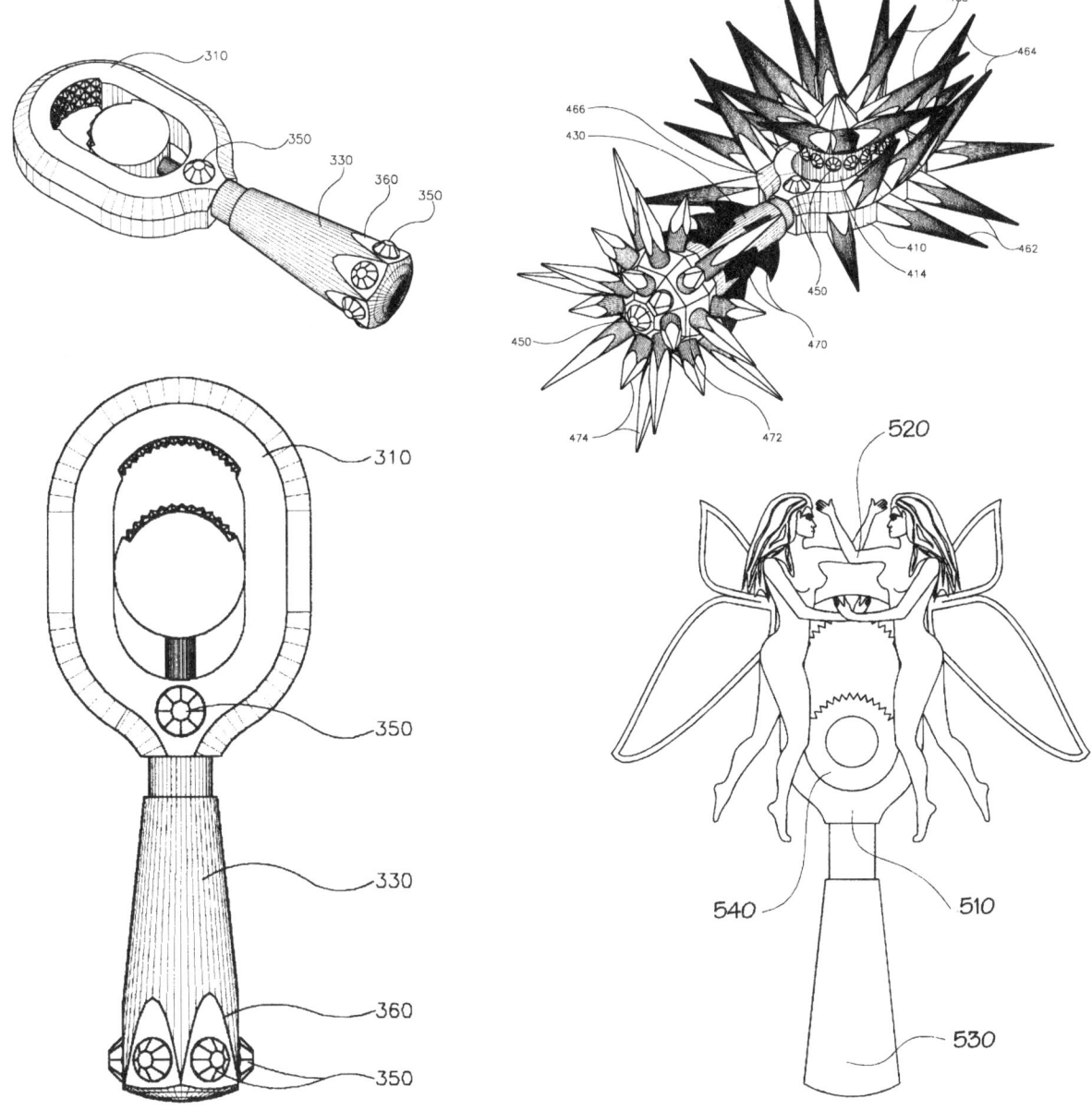

Patent No. 1,783,512
Dec 2, 1930
Mildred C. Mather

# Breast Protector

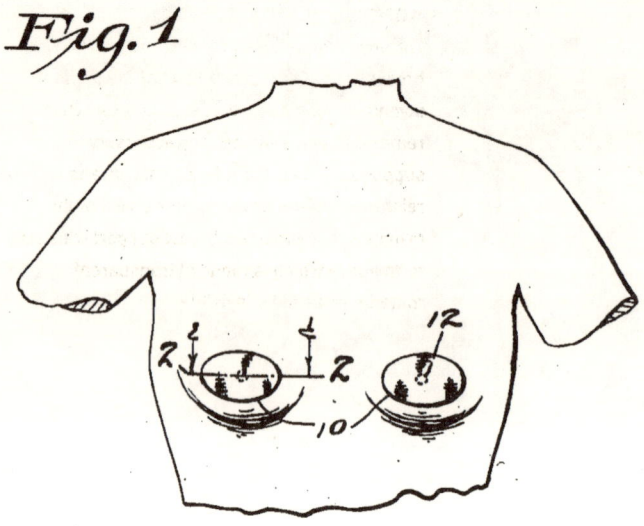

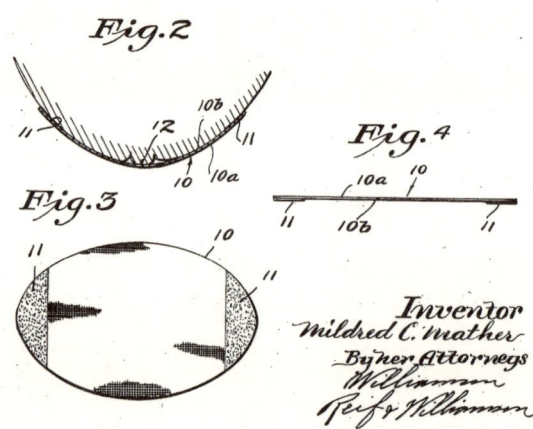

## Abstract

This invention relates to a breast protector or breast covering to be worn by girls and women. The present day tendency is for women, especially the younger women and girls, to wear few clothes, especially in the summertime. The brassiere or bandeaux commonly worn over the breasts is considered unnecessarily bulky by many girls who desire a lighter breast covering. It is desirable to have some covering over the breasts when wearing thin or tight fitting clothes, so that the nipples of the breast will not project unduly, and be too prominent or unsightly. Women and girls whose breasts are not greatly developed do not need any support therefore, and it is only necessary to have some means for rendering the nipple less prominent and conspicuous.

Patent No. 2,793,369
May 28, 1957
Franca Panighini

# Breast Supporter

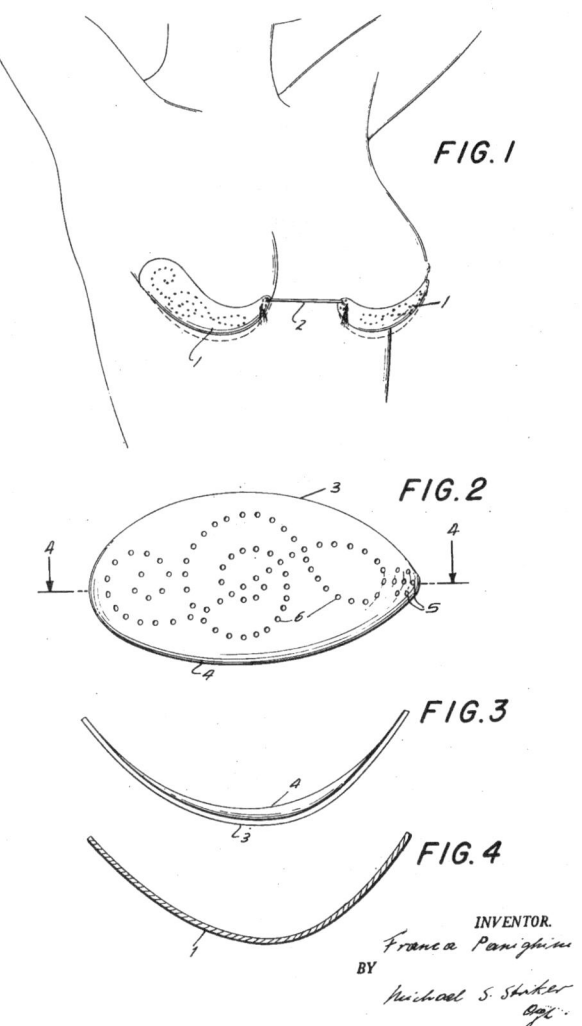

## Abstract

This invention relates to a new and improved breast supporter. It is an object of the present invention to provide a breast supporter which remains in place without any accessory supports such as shoulder or back straps or reinforcing members. A further object of the invention is to provide a breast supporter as set forth above which is made of transparent material so as to be invisible.

Patent No. US 6,338,344 B1
Jan 15, 2002
Andres Sinohui Jr.

# Chair Device for Enhancing Sexual Intimacy

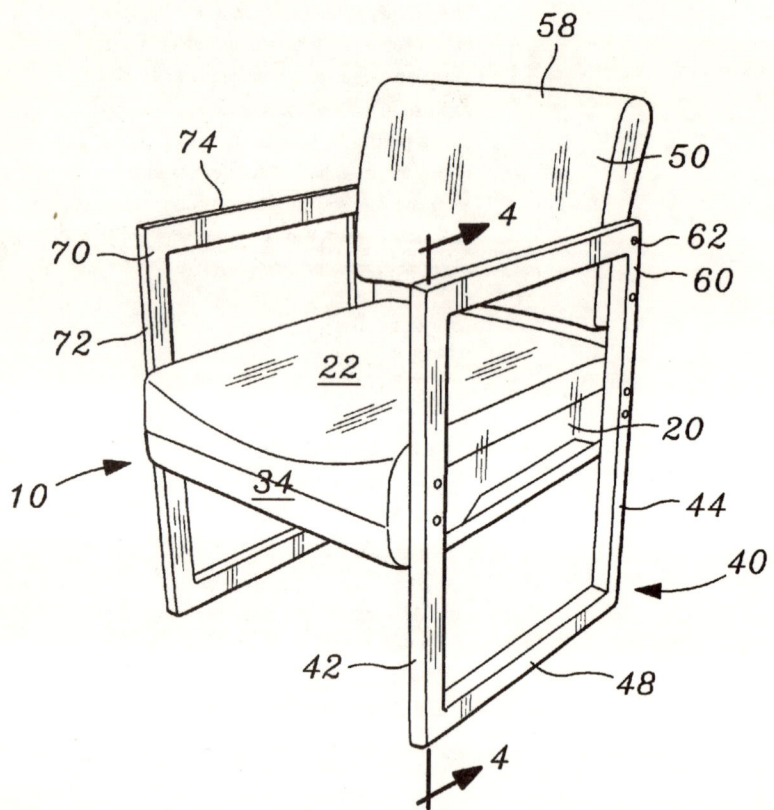

## Abstract

A chair device for facilitating sexual intimacy between a person and his or her sexual partner has a base attached to a back support frame and four legs. The chair device closely resembles and functions as an ordinary chair when resting in an upright position on its legs. When the chair device is turned over to an inverted position, the chair device is supported by the back support frame and an arm supporting means. In this inverted position, the base provides a padded reclining surface for supporting a person in a position that facilitates sexual intimacy with a sexual partner.

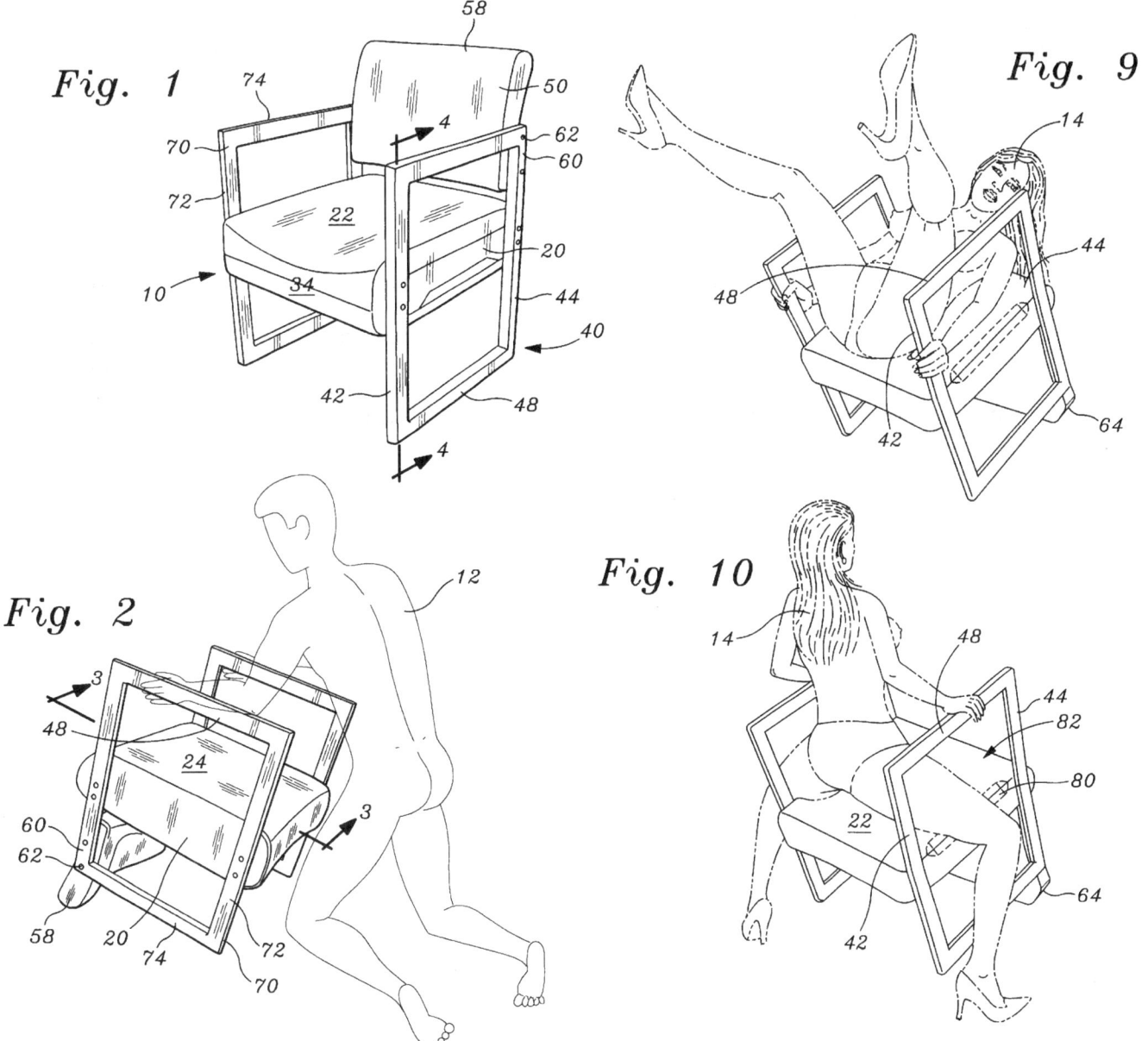

Patent No. US 6,520,906 B2
Feb 18, 2003
Senji Yanagi

# Coitus Assistance Device for Males

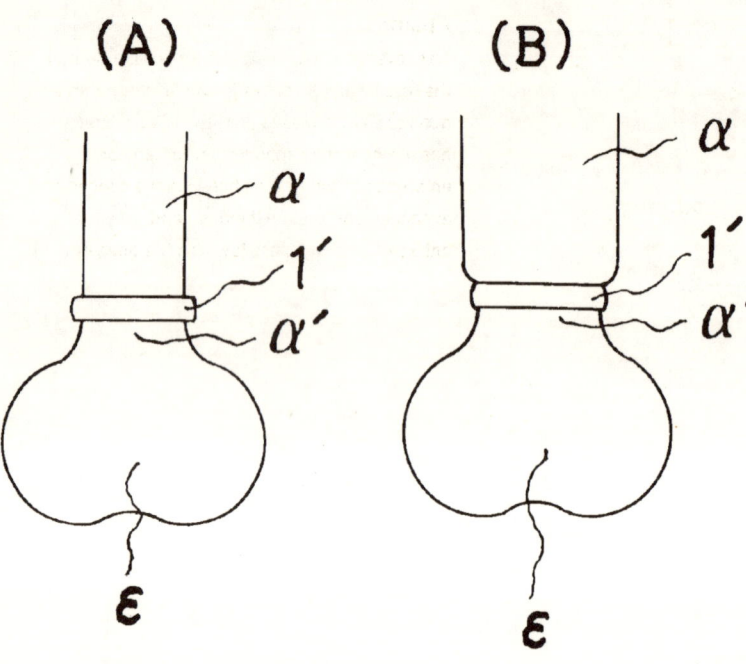

## Abstract

A gold band having a length normally required and width as normally required is flexible such that the gold band can be freely bent inward to form an oval ring of dimensions as normally required to oppress the root part of the inserted penis enlarged by erection. The gold band includes overlapping portions at opposed ends thereof which are overlapped to form the oval ring. Patterned protrusions for oppressing the urogenital canal in the root part of the erect penis enlarged by erection are provided over a specified area at the entry of the inner surface of the gold band.

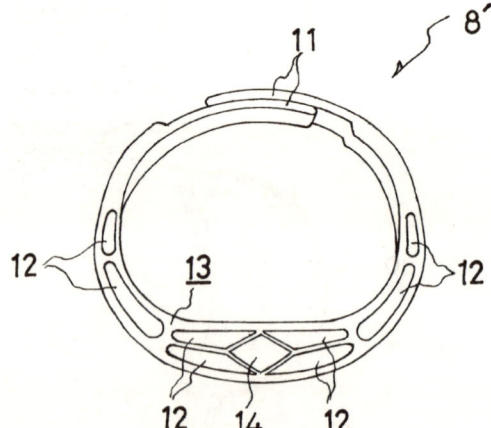

Patent No. 5,398,699
Mar 21, 1995
Thomas Fergus

# Condom

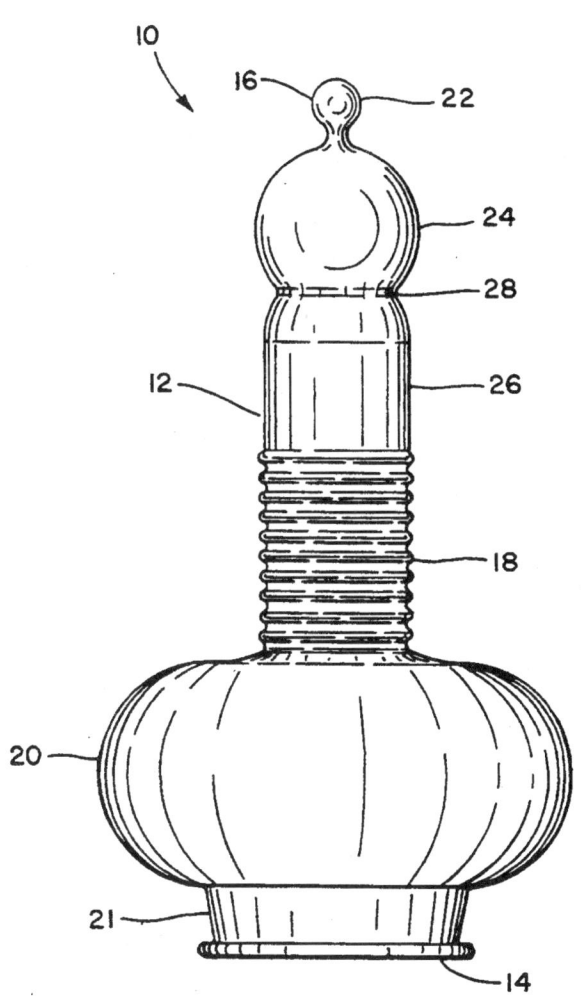

## Abstract

This invention provides an improved condom of the type having a generally tubular body with an open end and a closed end. The tubular body has a concertina expander portion and an enlarged portion located between the concertina expanded portion and the open end. The enlarged portion tapers towards the open end.

Patent No. 5,318,043
June 7, 1994
Lawrence S. Burr; Kenneth Matsumura

## Condom for Oral-Genital Use

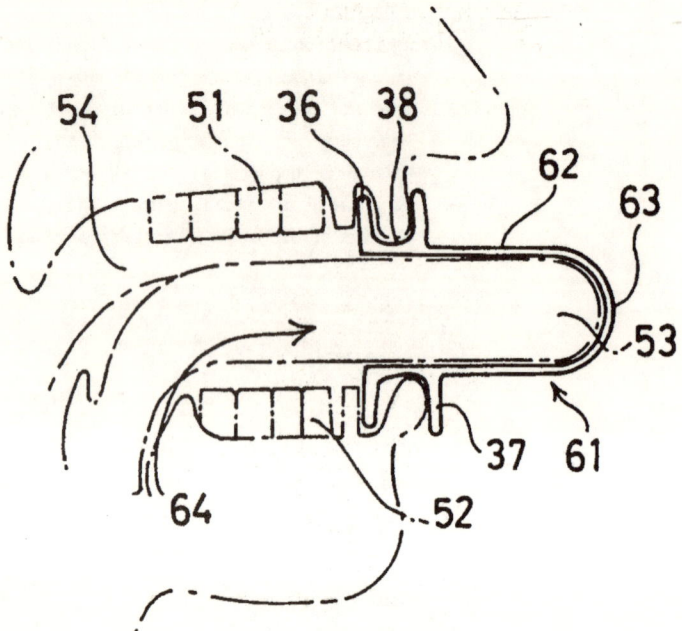

### Abstract

A condom designed for oral-genital sex includes, in one aspect, a device adapted to be worn in the mouth of the person practicing oral sex. The device includes a tubular member having one closed end and formed of thin, pliant, impervious material. Joined to the open end of the tubular member are two or three flanges extending generally radially outwardly and spaced closely together. The device is gripped by placing the lips within the channel, and closing the jaws slightly to compress and retain the open end of the device. The tubular member may be formed to extend into the mouth of the wearer, for the purpose of performing fellatio. A penis may be inserted into the tubular member without making contact with the lips or mouth or tongue of the wearer. The flange is provided with means for engaging and sealing with the outer circumferential edge portion of a typical prior art male condom, so that the shield may be joined temporarily to a commercially available condom for the practice of safe sex.

FIG. 7

FIG. 8

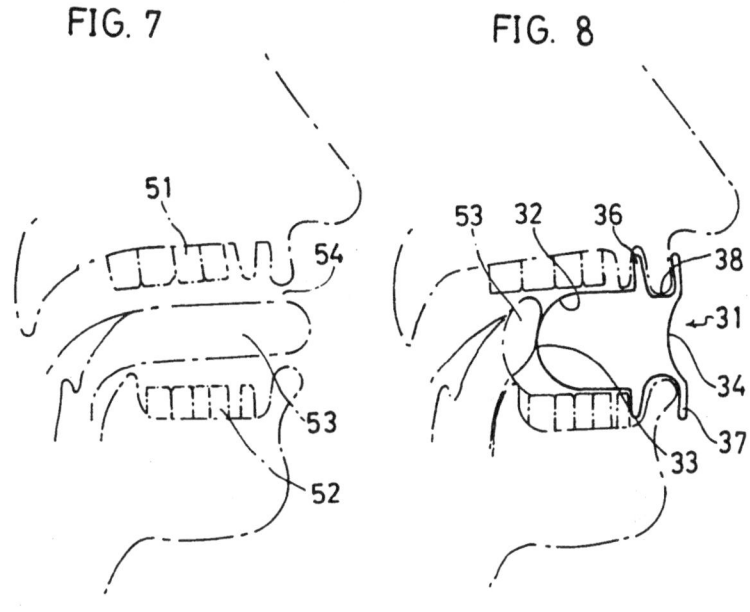

FIG. 9

FIG. 10

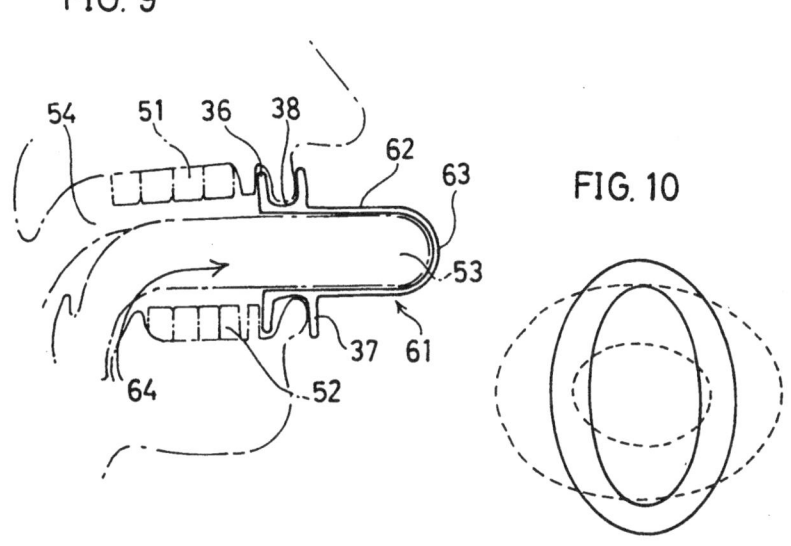

Patent No. 6,098,626
Aug 8, 2000
Hye-Sook Kim

# Condom with Multi-Purpose Sexual Device

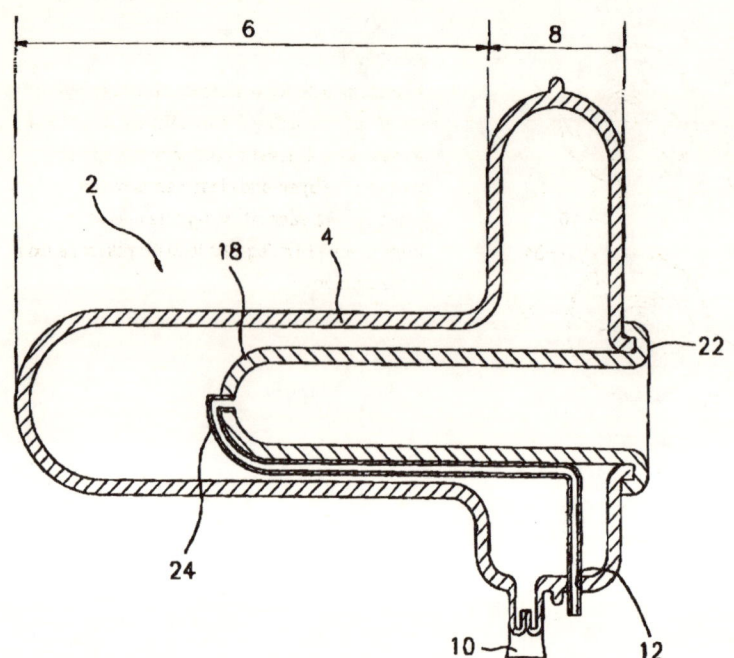

## Abstract

This invention relates to a condom having a hard case, an air hole formed at one side of an outer sheet at a rear end of the condom, and a tube for maintaining atmospheric pressure in the hard case and connecting the air hole with a nose of the hard case, the tube is located in an air inflation chamber which is defined by the hard case and said outer sheet thus the condom to perfecting not only contraception and preventing venereal disease but also aiding other sexual problems such as premature ejaculation and insufficient erection.

# Condom with Spiral Crisscross Ribbing

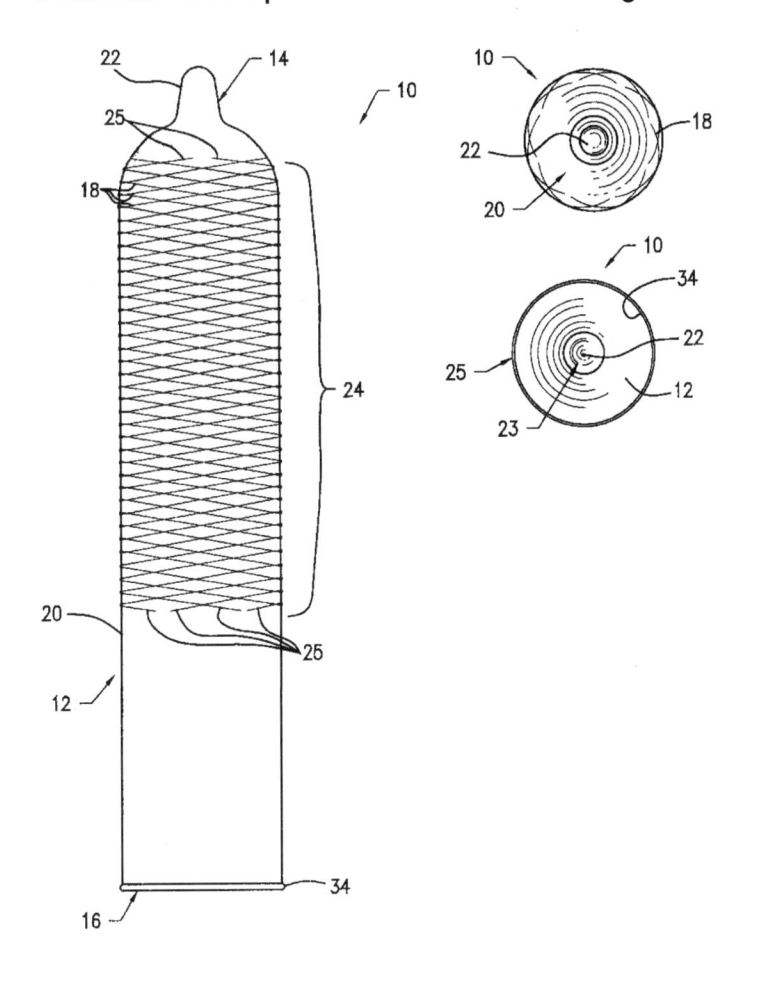

Patent No. US 6,321,751 B1
Nov 27, 2001
Steven R. Strauss; Richard D. Kline;
Jim D. Burns; Michael J. Harrison

## Abstract

A condom includes a plurality of intersecting spiral ribs extending in two different directional planes along at least a portion of the surface between the open and closed ends of the condom, with each rib being oriented at an angle of about 15 degrees to the transverse axis of the condom.

Patent No. 4,971,071
Nov 20, 1990
Gary D. Johnson

# Conductive Condom

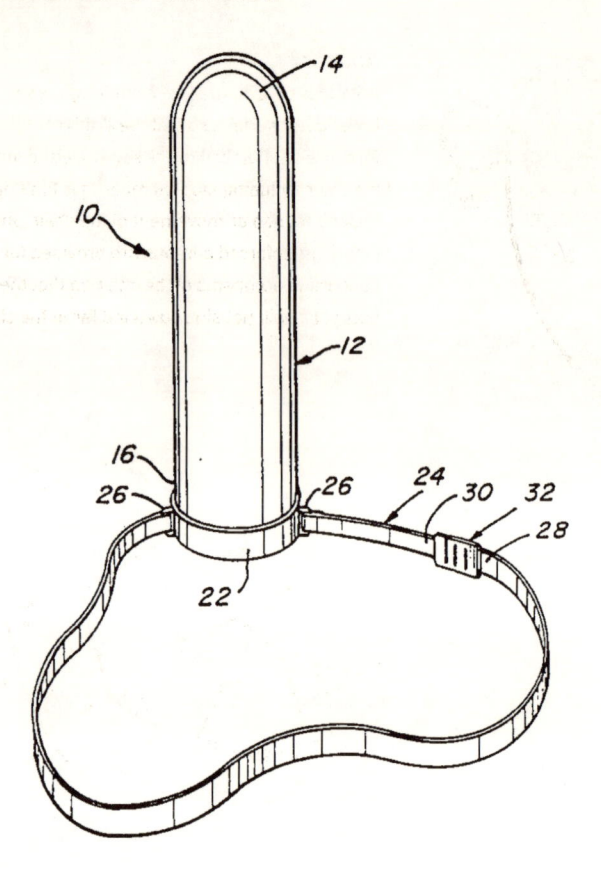

## Abstract

An electrically conductive condom includes a generally cylindrical protective sheath having an open end for receiving a penis therein and an opposite closed end, the sheath being made from a thin, elastic, electrically conductive material which may be formed from a non-conductive elastic material having electrically conductive particles embedded therein. Optionally, a retaining strap may be secured to the reinformcing layer for retaining the sheath on a person.

Patent No. 4,099,773
July 11, 1978
James F. Chang

# Couple's Chair

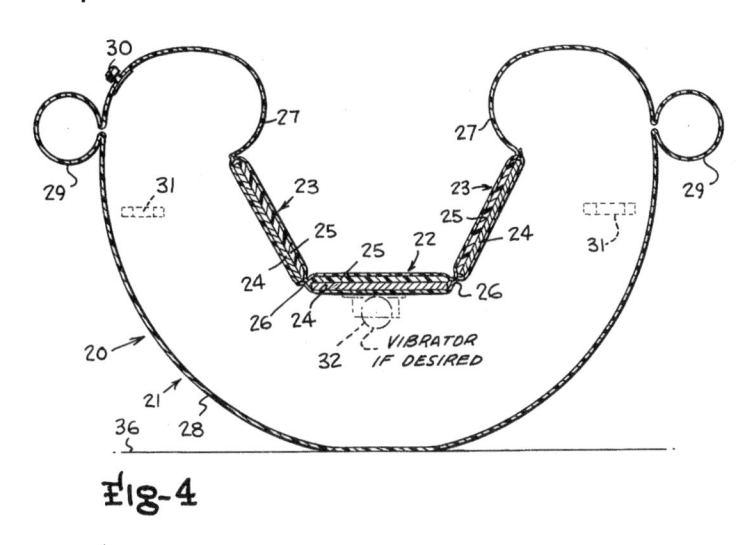

## Abstract

An article of furniture that includes a curved lower outer surface so that the article of furniture or chair can be rocked back and forth, the chair including stop members for limiting rocking motion or movement of the chair, and wherein reinforced portions are provided for supporting occupants of the chair so that the occupants will not sink down too far in the chair.

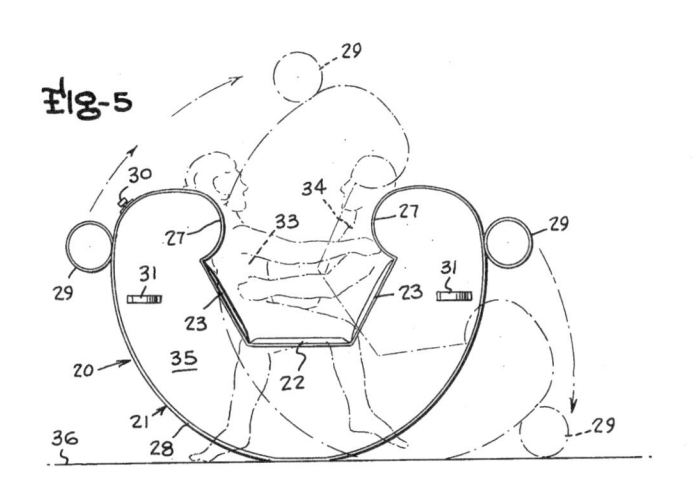

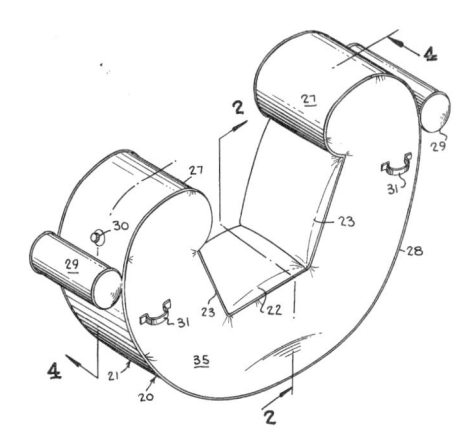

# Decorative Penile Wrap

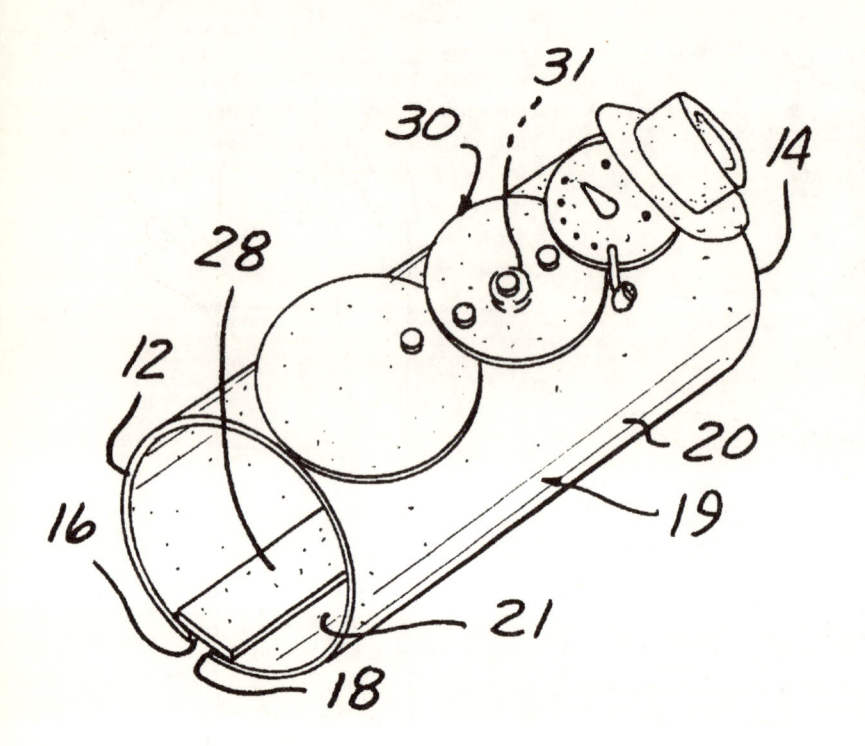

Patent No. 6,145,506
Nov 14, 2000
Dawn M. Goll

## Abstract

A decorative penile wrap encircles a human male penis. The decorative penile wrap is in the form of a cylindrical sheath having a hollow interior and opposed, open, first and second ends. A fastener is provided in one embodiment for securing opposed side edges of the sheath together to form a planar sheet into a cylindrical sheath. Decorative indicia is formed on the exterior of the sheath to provide a stimulating appearance. Alternately, the sheath is formed with a continuous, closed side wall.

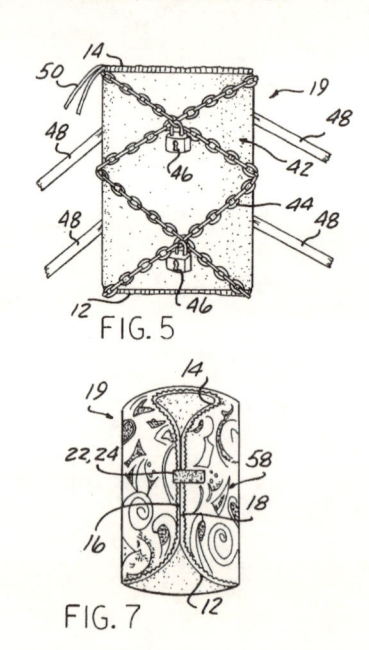

FIG. 5

FIG. 7

FIG. 9

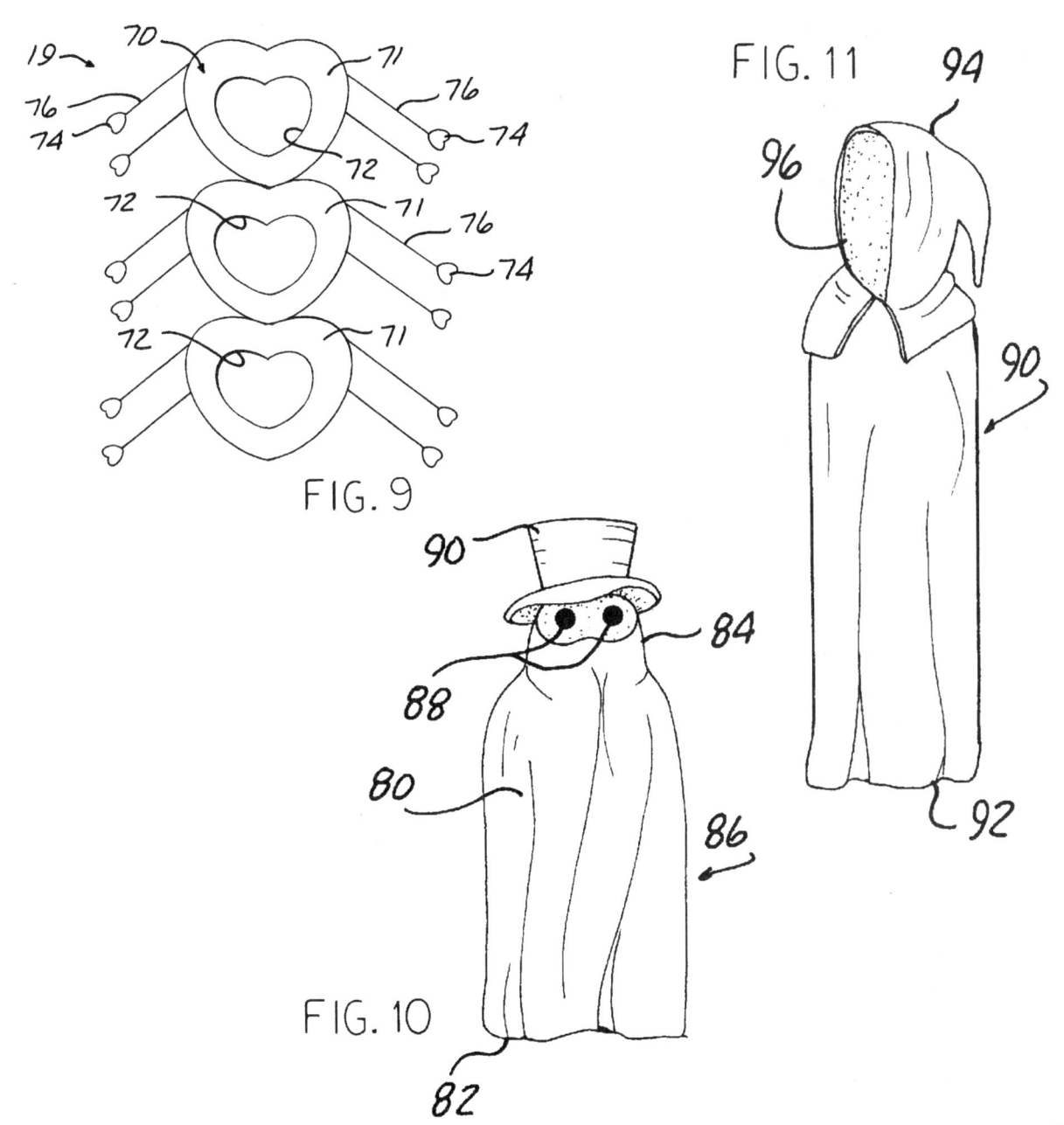

FIG. 11

FIG. 10

Patent No. 4,643,175
Feb 17, 1987
Kenneth Chapman

# Device for Assisting and Maintaining an Erection

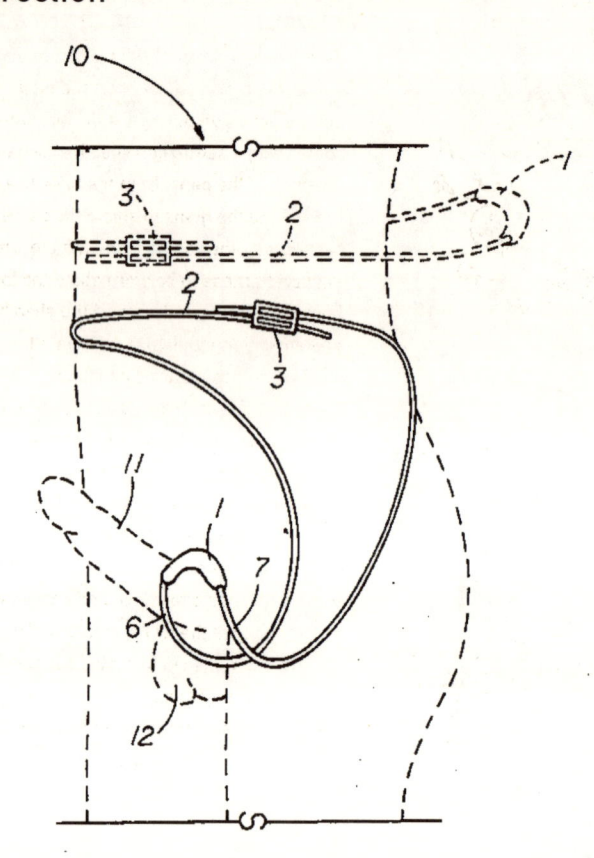

## Abstract
A device for assisting in and maintaining erection of the human penis, comprising: a relatively rigid arc member and an elastic cord extending from each end of the arc member and joined to form a large loop.

Patent No. 4,381,000
Apr 26, 1983
Lee G. Duncan

# Device for Use in Human Copulation

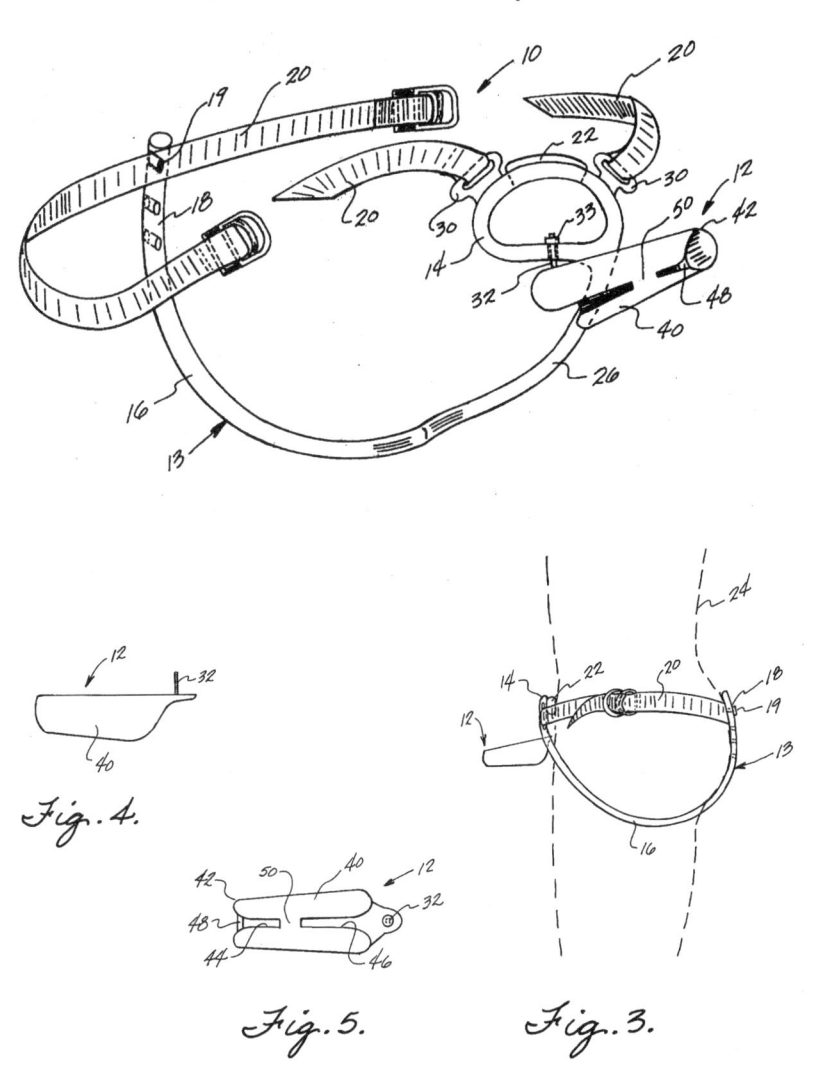

## Abstract

A device to be worn by the human male during sexual intercourse to support the penis and delay ejaculation during the act of copulation, comprising a semi-rigid sheath which encircles the shaft of the penis from the base to a point just behind the glans to shield the same from contact with the vagina of the female, and a support harness to be worn about the lower body of the male and support the sheath to prevent its longitudinal movement along the shaft of the penis during copulation. The harness includes an elongate semi-rigid section having a base portion which is located centrally on the lower abdomen of the male above the penis to firmly engage the pubic bone, and a semi-rigid member which extends from the base portion through the crotch area of the wearer and has a terminal end portion which firmly engages the lower vertebra of the spine to form a dimensionally stable support for the penis-encircling sheath. Strap means are provided for securing the semi-rigid support section of the harness to the body of the wearer.

Patent No. US 6,179,775 B1
Jan 30, 2001
Ronald J. Thompson

# Device to Enhance Clitoral Stimulation During Intravaginal Intercourse

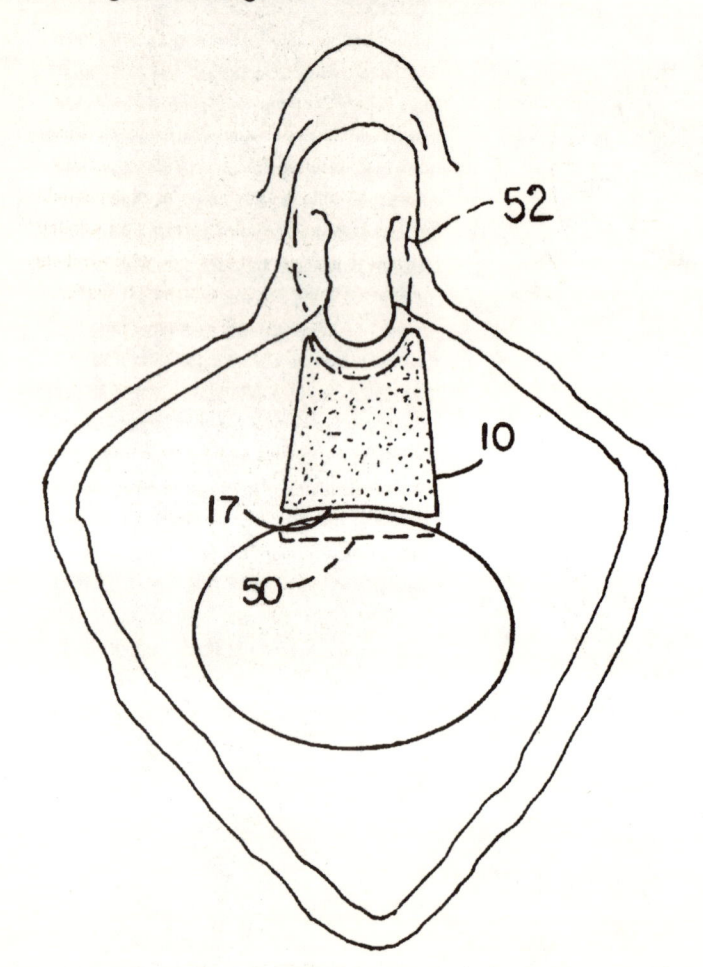

## Abstract

The present invention includes an apparatus for the increased female clitoral stimulation. The apparatus comprises a foraminous, elongated, generally triangularly shaped pad having an anterior portion arranged to support and engage the ventral aspect of the clitoris and lie beneath the labia minora. The pad has an outer peripheral contour so as to seat within the female vestibule. The pad is comprised of a plurality of layers of flexible material. The pad has an uppermost layer of soft flexible material and an intermediate layer of generally semi-rigid material and a lower layer of an adhesive material.

Patent No. 2,869,553
Jan 20, 1959
Nici D'Or

# Disposable Tear-Away Brassiere

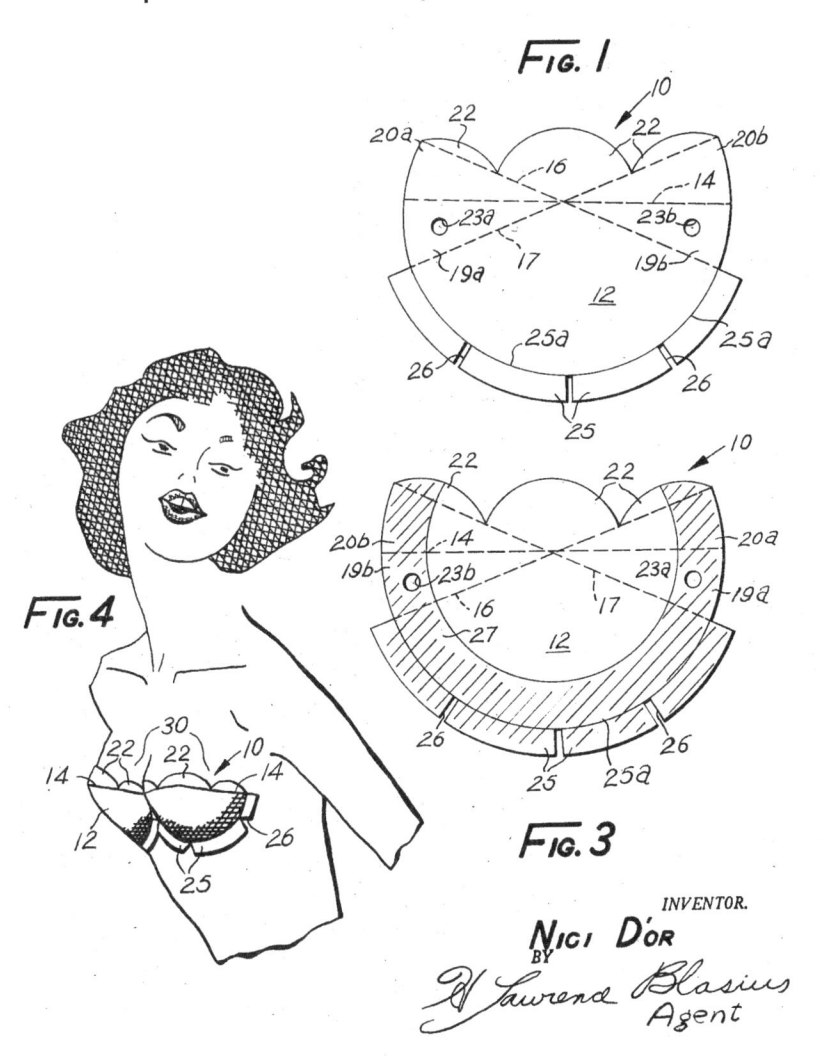

## Abstract

This invention relates to garments and more particularly to a brassiere. Because the straps are unsightly and shoulder straps cannot be worn with summer wear and low neck dresses, and also because the back straps especially are uncomfortable to wear and are not dependable, efforts have been made to provide a so-called strapless brassiere, that is, one which will stay in place without the use of straps. It has for example been proposed to apply them adhesively by employing pressure sensitive adhesive around the breast cups and thus make them self sustaining. However such articles, however supported, do not function to lift up the breasts and support them in elevated position which is desirable both for hygienic reasons and for the sake of appearance.

43

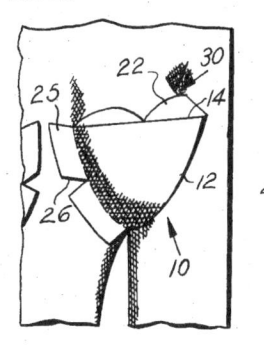

Patent No. 5,655,543
Aug 12, 1997
Paula A. Bloodsaw

# Ear Fastener for Oral Condoms

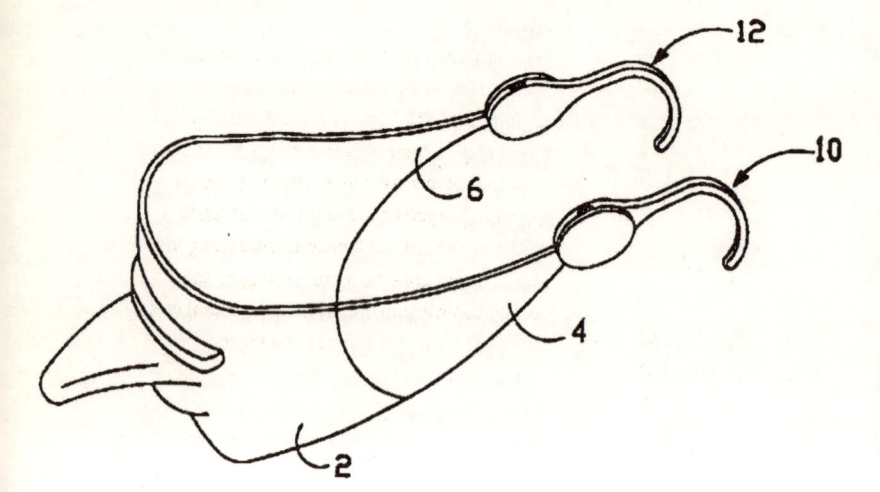

## Abstract

An ear fastener used in conjunction with an oral condom which protects the user from contracting sexually transmitted diseases while engaging in cunnilingus and anal sex. The ear fastener facilitates the clamping and releasing of the lateral end of the oral condom. The ear fastener has a front clamping portion, a rear engagement portion for partially engaging over and behind an ear of a user, and a cover hingeably connected to the front portion by a living hinge. The cover can be hingeably opened or closed such that a central protruding pin aligns with and snaps in a central protruding socket provided on the proximal portion for securing and clamping the lateral end of the oral condom.

Patent No. 609,614
Aug 23, 1898
James Doty

# Electrical Appliance for Assisting Anatomical Organs

Fig. 1.

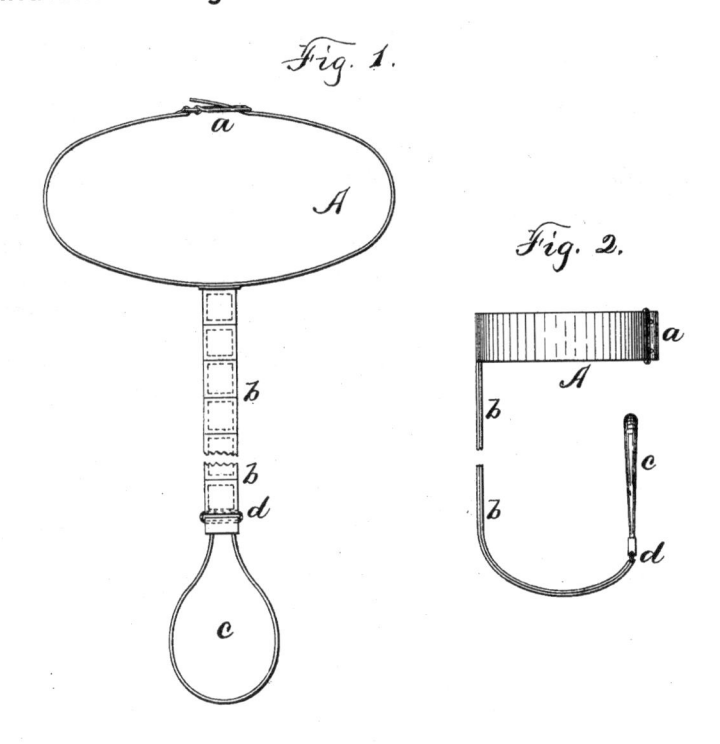

Fig. 2.

WITNESSES:

INVENTOR
James Doty

## Abstract

My invention relates to devices and appliances for assisting anatomical organs in the performance of inherent natural functions. The object of my invention is to produce an improved appliance of this class whereby the male generative organs are aided and enabled to perform their natural functions, consisting in an elastic device creating a pressure upon the corpus cavernosum and against the crural roots in front of the pelvis and passing behind the scrotum, combined with suitable means for producing a longitudinal strain upon said device to increase or regulate its tensional pressure, such as an electric belt or a connection to and in circuit with such a belt, whereby the electromagnetic power applied strength is given to the branches of the pubic nerves and the hypogastric plexus and the muscles are stimulated to a complete condition, the loop being wholly elastic and when drawn tight elastically bears against the upper side of the organ, producing a congestion and holding the blood confined in the erectile tissue for a sufficient length of time.

# Electromechanical Massager Apparatus

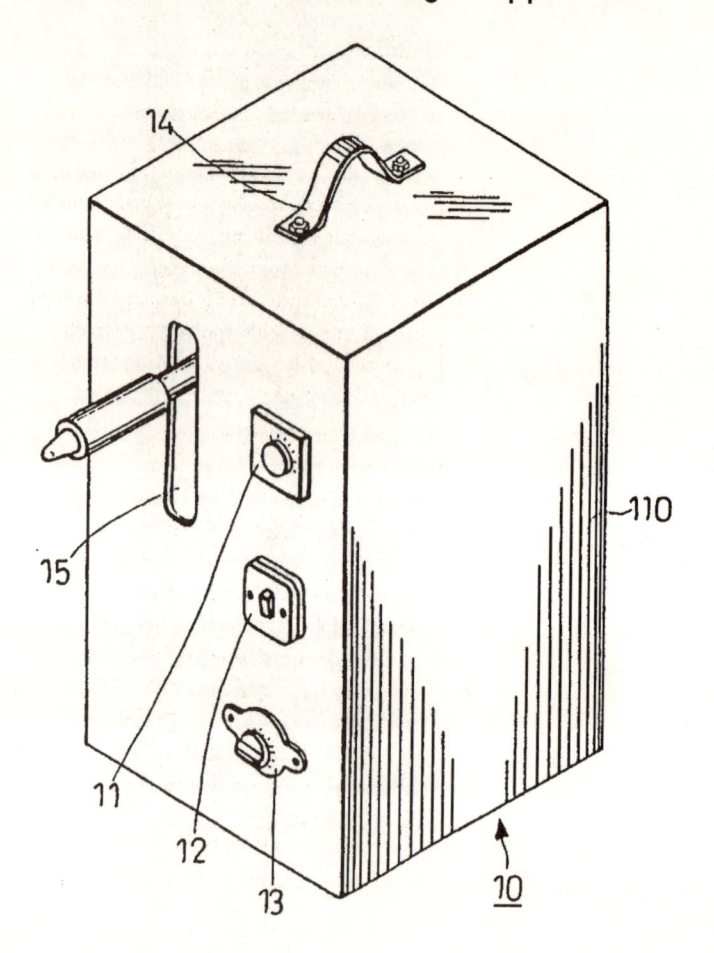

Patent No. 4,834,075
May 30, 1989
Yuh-Kuen Guo; Feng-Mei Song

## Abstract

An electromechanical massage apparatus including a massage body structure and a detachable supporting mount wherein the massage body structure includes a housing unit adapted to be positioned on a place adjacent to the detachable supporting mount and provided with a speed regulator, a switch and a timer on a front side of the housing unit. The detachable supporting mount includes: a plurality of partitioning boards with different binding straps vertically disposed on top of the supporting place for supporting a portion of a human body so as to perform massage operations.

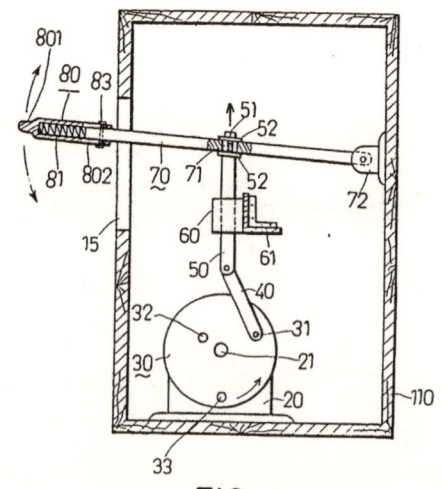

FIG. 2

Patent No. 4,240,413
Dec 23, 1980
Judith Hanus

# Erection Holder

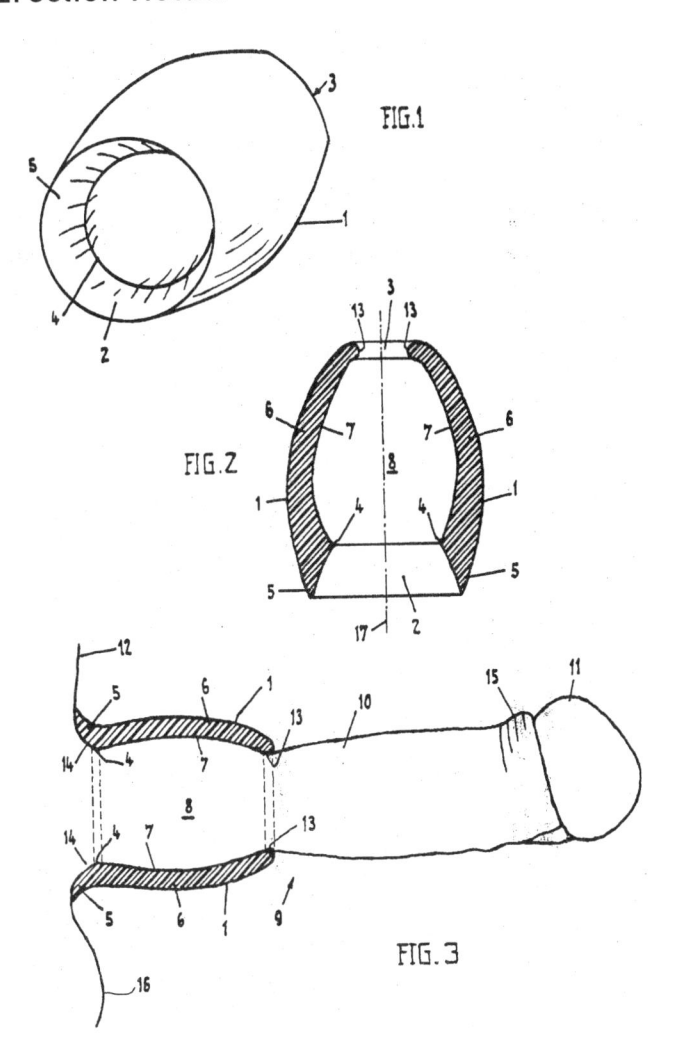

## Abstract

An erection holder to enable or prolong an erection of the penis of a man. It has a body of sleeve-like configuration with an outer sleeve wall surface, a hollow interior surrounded by an inner sleeve wall surface, a base end destined for coming to rest, during use, against a portion of the user's abdomen, surrounding the root of his penis, and an outer end. Openings are in the base end and the inner end. A first inwardly directed protrusion surrounds the opening in the base end and a second inwardly directed protrusion surrounds the opening in the outer end.

# Erogenic Stimulator

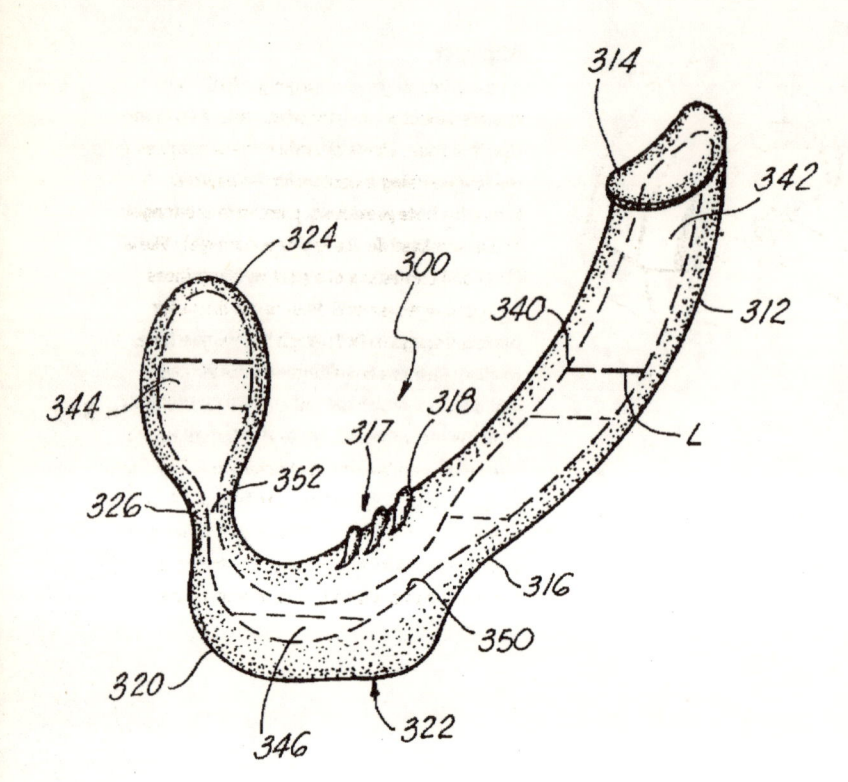

Patent No. 5,690,603
Nov 25, 1997
Melissa Mia Kain

## Abstract

A self-retaining erogenic stimulator that provides simultaneous stimulation to both users thereof, whether they be of the same sex or of the opposite sex. This stimulator is configured with a first phallic end which is used in the normal manner and a second bulbous end which is inserted within the vaginal or anal cavity of the wearing partner. This bulbous end is shaped with a neck-down region that enables this device to be held in place during use by the wearers' muscle groups without the need for straps or the like. Also, adjacent to the base of the phallic end may be raised nubs which are designed for the clitoral stimulation of the wearing partner (when such partner is female) whether the device is inserted vaginally or anally. A hollowed-out area in the base can hold vibrating means for increased stimulation; or a fluid chamber within the apparatus allows the flow of fluid therein to increase stimulation.

Patent No. US 6,419,649 B1
July 16, 2002
Eric A. Klein

# Erotic Stimulation Device (Tongue Roller)

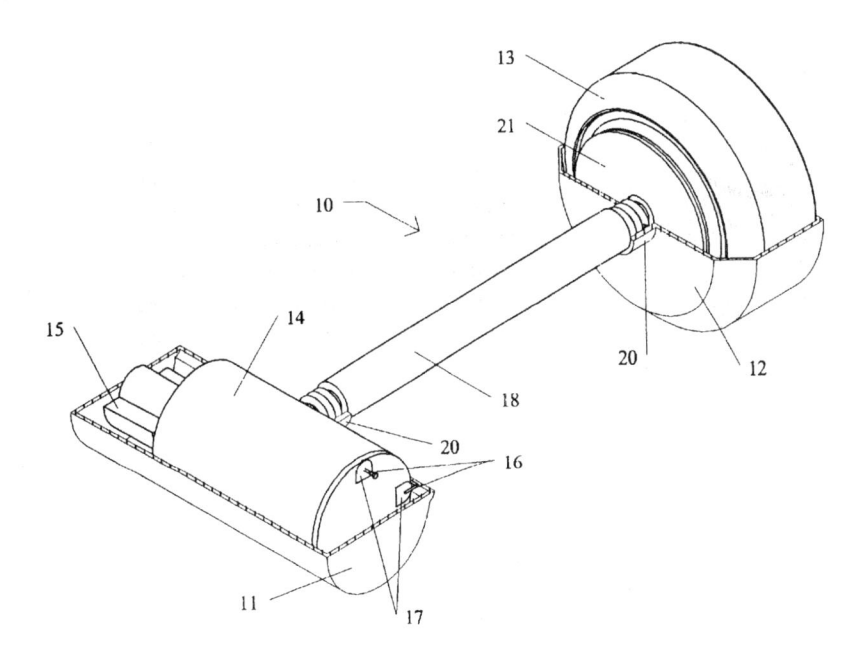

## Abstract

A sexual aid device comprising a battery powered electric vibrator which attaches to the user's tongue. The first embodiment attaches to the tongue using a post which is inserted through a hole previously pierced in the tongue. The assembled device is shaped roughly like a dumbbell consisting of a post with retainers mounted at either end. Post has a diameter narrow enough to fit through the tongue hole, but the retainers have larger diameter and cannot slip through the hole. An electric vibrator motor is incorporated into one of the retainers. The second embodiment attaches to the tongue using suction, constriction, and friction. A pliable plastic mouthpiece is mounted at the rear of the device. The interior of mouthpiece forms a tongue cup into which the user inserts the tongue.

Patent No. 5,657,765
Aug 19, 1997
Steven S. Est

# Erotic Stimulator

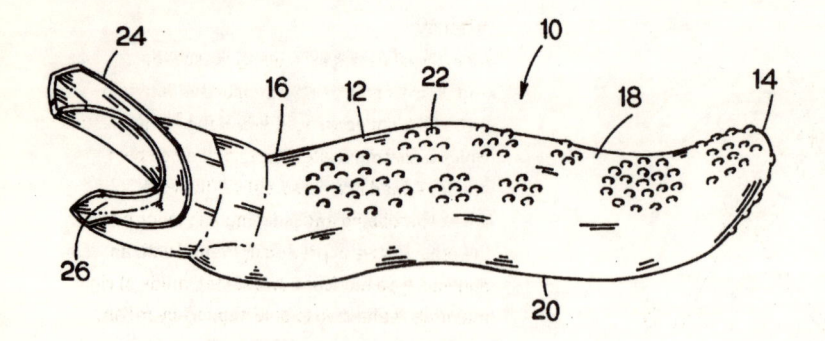

## Abstract

An erotic stimulator in the form of a tongue is provided. The stimulator comprises a flexible, elongated member having a mouthpiece at its base end whereby a user can manipulate the stimulator while leaving the hands free during gynecological stimulation with the device. The device has a plurality of raised projections on its surface to provide enhanced stimulation to the more sensitive areas of the female anatomy.

Patent No. 5,928,134
July 27, 1999
Roberto Jose Romero Vergara

# External Device for Eluding Masculine Impotence

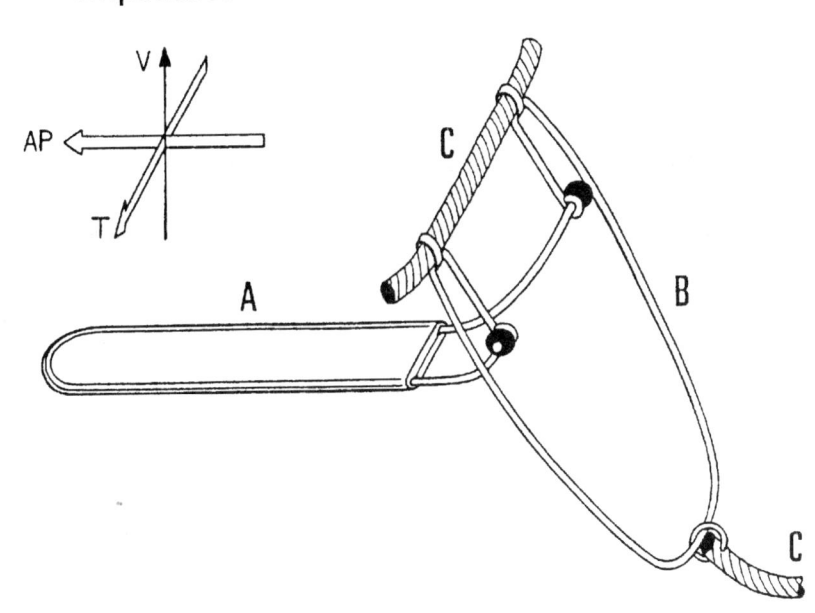

## Abstract

An external device for eluding masculine impotence, comprising a support, with a rigid core and a softer lining, it lies along the penis, to which it communicates its rigidity, since both are enveloped in a preservative. To avoid tautness, rubbing and pinching, the inner side of the preservative is previously wetted with an aqueous type lubricant. A fastener, made of rigid material, is attached to said support by means of two hinges, thus maintaining the support in its proper place despite the effort exerted during its use. It is useful for coitus performance when the erection is nonexistent or insufficient in intensity of duration.

Patent No. 5,842,970
Dec 1, 1998
Ronald J. Lakusiewicz

# External Penile Prosthetic Device

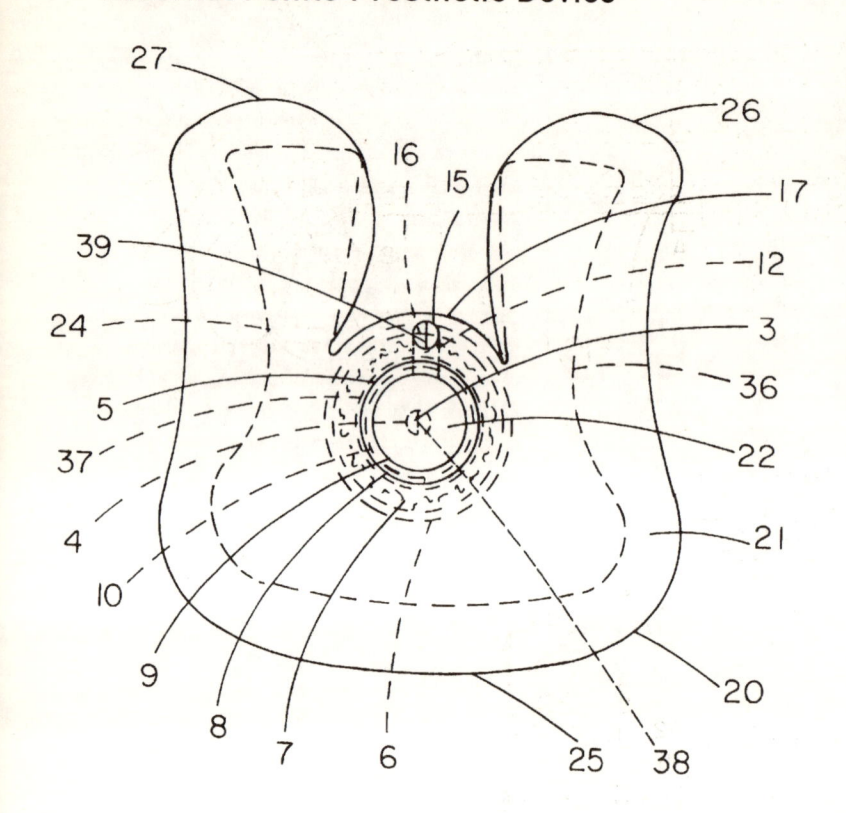

## Abstract

An external penile prosthetic device is adapted to be worn on the groin and suprapubic areas of the wearer. The device has a generally tubular outer wall made from a flexible material, having an open proximal end and a closed distal end, the exterior of the outer wall being configured to resemble an erect human penis. A viscous fluid fills the chamber between the outer wall and the inner wall. A flange is disposed around and connected to the proximal end of the outer wall of the prosthetic device for mounting the device over the groin and suprapubic areas of the wearer.

FIG. 1

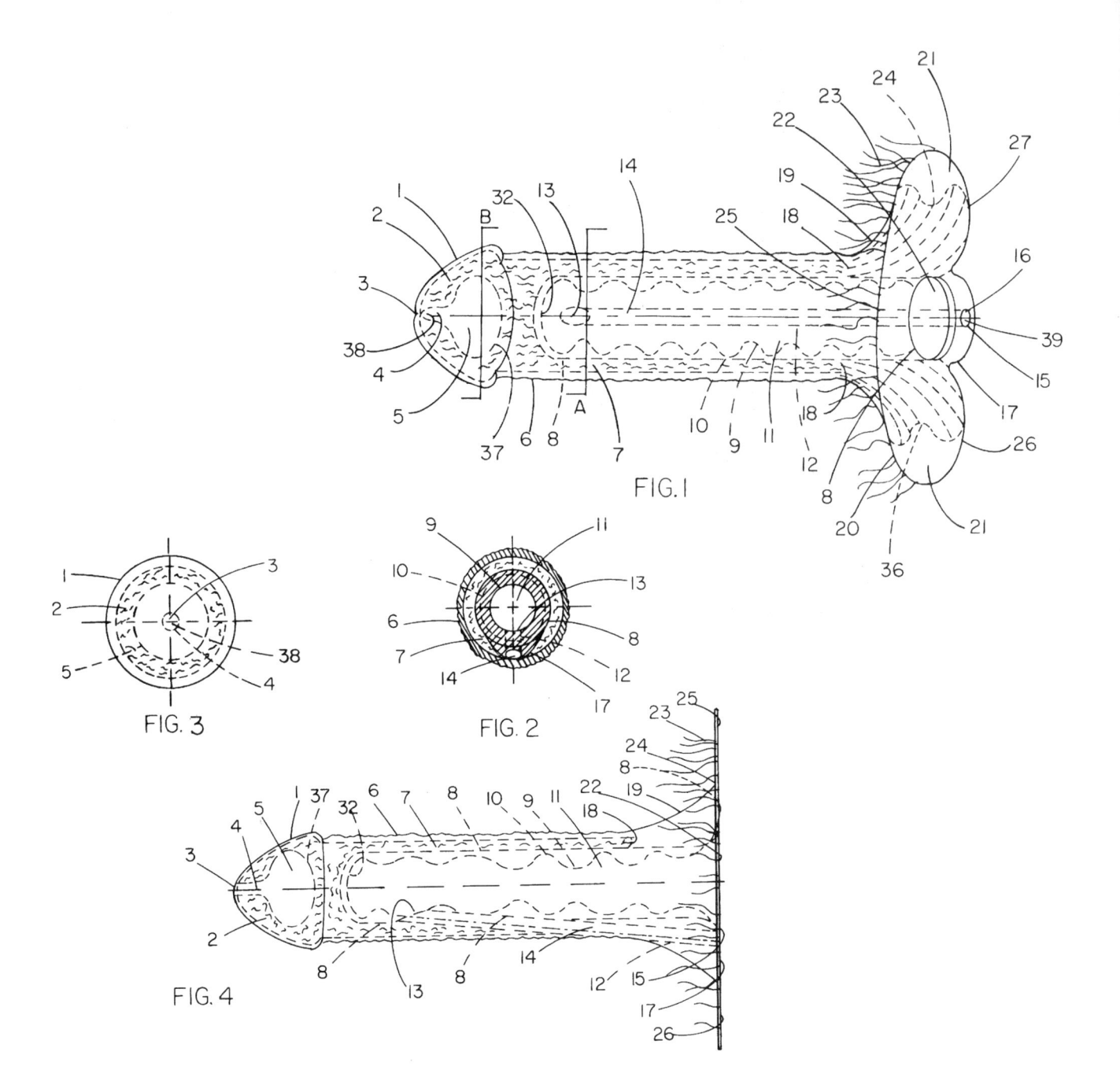

FIG. 3

FIG. 2

FIG. 4

Patent No. US 6,436,029 B1
Aug 20, 2002
Theodore V. Benderev

# External Vibratory Exercising Device for Pelvic Muscles

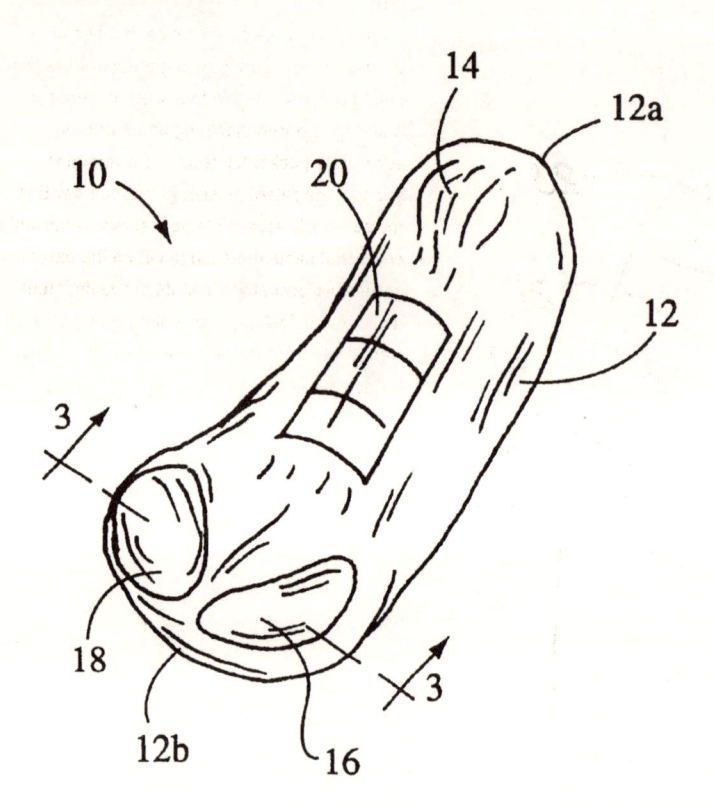

## Abstract

A device and method for treating urinary as well as fecal incontinence by selectively and controllably imparting stimuli to the pelvic region. The device is adapted to be compressively positioned against the crotch of the user to thus identify target pelvic floor muscles and muscle groups responsible for urinary and/or fecal continence and provide periodic stimulus thereto by way of pressure, stretching, resistance, vibration, and/or heat. The device may be further utilized to impart magnetic therapy to the pelvic region of the user or may include a stimulator for imparting a pleasurable sensation to the sex organs.

# Female Condom

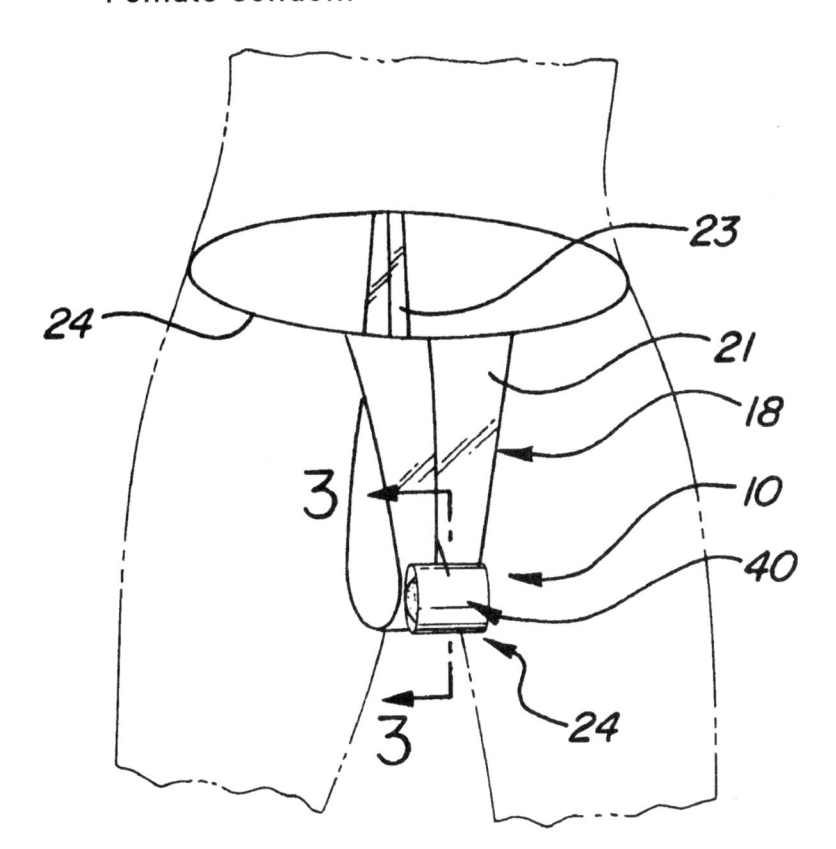

Patent No. 6,035,853
Mar 14, 2000
Ravikumar Alla; Madhusudhan Alla; Raghunatha Alla

## Abstract

A female condom has a pouch that has a predeployment position on the outer surface of a shield portion wherein the pouch includes a telescoped portion forming an exteriorly accessible pocket for receiving a retention sponge; the retention sponge is sealed within the exteriorly accessible pocket by a removable cover that seals the sponge within the exteriorly accessible pocket while in its predeployment position, the locking and sealing member is removable from the telescoped pouch portion for deployment.

Patent No. 5,285,531
Feb 15, 1994
Robert M. Nalbandian

# Female Garment

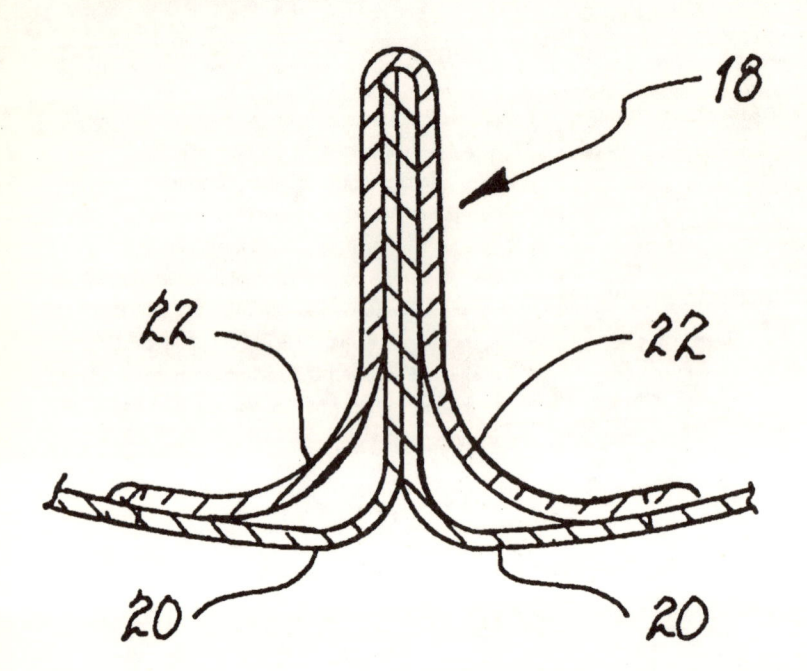

### Abstract

The present invention provides a female garment with an infolding or cleft at the surface level of the labia majora to subtly define the contours of the external female genitalia. The features of the external female genitalia in situ may be represented in a variety of female garments by utilizing first and second layers where the first layer constitutes material of the female garment and the second layer constitutes material of a different color or texture from that of the first material.

Fig. 1

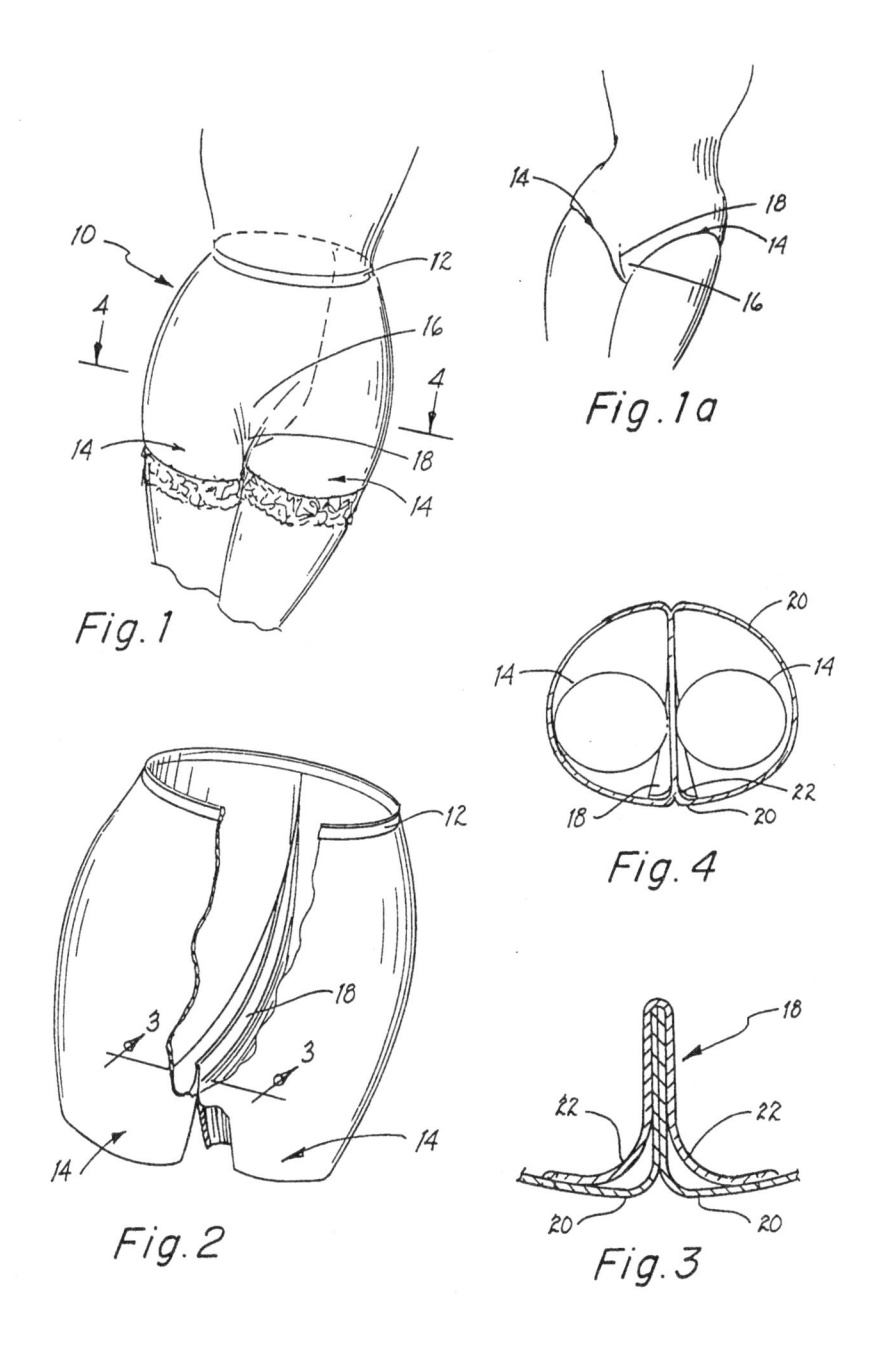

Fig. 1a

Fig. 2

Fig. 3

Fig. 4

Patent No. 6,099,463
Aug 8, 2000
Robert Hockhalter

# Female Stimulator Comprising Close-Fitting Clitoral Suction Chamber

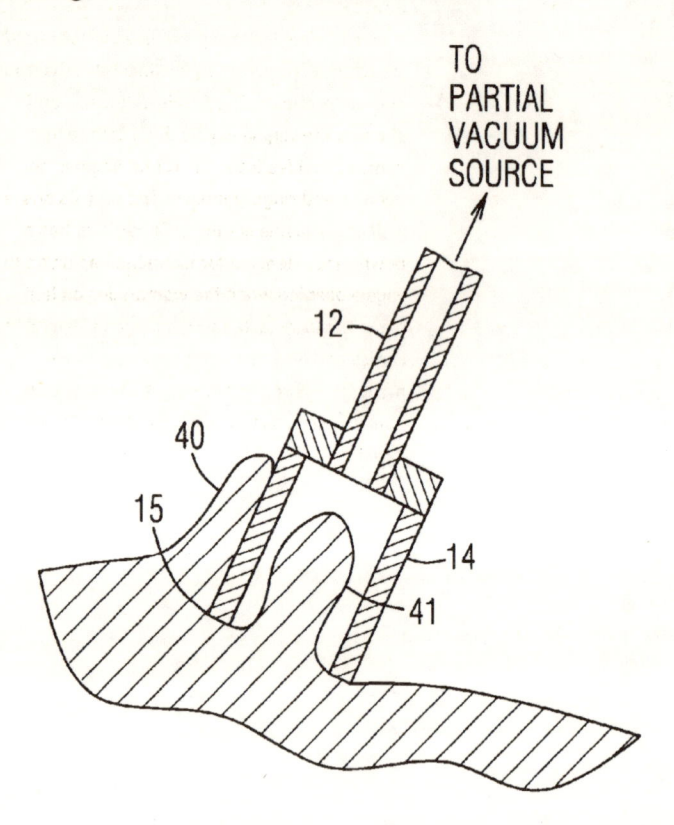

## Abstract

A female stimulation device is comprised of a tubular suction chamber sized for closely fitting around a clitoris. The suction chamber is connected to a variable partial vacuum source through a tubing. The partial vacuum source may be the mouth of a user or a mechanical device, such as a vacuum bulb or pump. The clitoris is drawn outwardly by the partial vacuum, so that it is engorged with blood to produce a sexually pleasurable sensation. The force of suction may be controlled by a check and suction release valve, which is also used to release the partial vacuum. The front end of the suction chamber is shaped to provide an airtight but comfortable seal.

Patent No. 5,620,429
Apr 15, 1997
Abdul A. A. Al-Saleh

# Feminine Napkin Allows External Sexual Intercourse

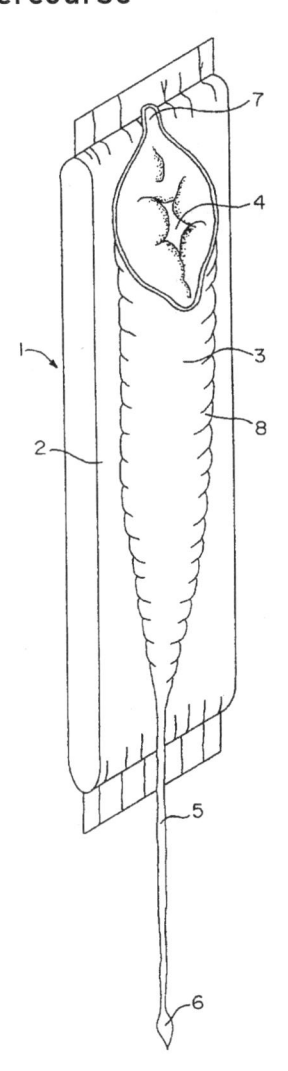

## Abstract

A feminine napkin that permits external sexual intercourse. A round bag is attached to the front side of the napkin. The bag is in the size and shape of the vagina to give the husband the same sexual feelings. The round bag has an opening and rings, windings and protrusions, as well as a suitable cream. This bag also has a downward extension for fixing the napkin on the vagina opening when the woman lies on her back. The fixing extension is placed between the rumps and may be coated by an adhesive material. The round bag can be taken off the napkin and disposed while continuing to use the napkin.

Patent No. 5,853,362
Dec 29, 1998
Deborah A. Jacobs

# Glandular Stimulator Device and Method

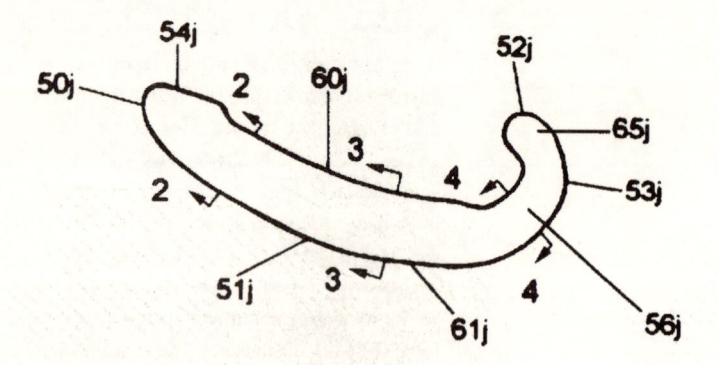

## Abstract

An intravaginal glandular stimulator device is sized and shaped to be worn internally by a woman. That is, a predetermined hook shaped device constructed of sufficiently rigid material is provided so that the proximal end of the device rests in a vaginal subcavity adjacent to the woman's Grafenberg spot. The proximal end is shaped and angled to exert pressure against the Grafenberg spot, and to resist dislodgement except by conscious muscular relaxation and manual pulling. The stimulator's extravaginal or distal end may be shaped like a dildo to be used for vaginally or anally penetrating a partner; shaped recumbently upon itself and used to stimulate the external genitalia of the wearer; or shaped as a handle to be manipulated by the wearer or by her partner. The stimulator provides an easy-to-affix shape for sexual stimulation of the wearer without the necessity of straps, buckles, or the like; and provides a predetermined hook curvature for genital-to-genital sexual contact between two female partners in positions not otherwise possible. It further allows for simultaneous Grafenberg spot and prostate gland stimulation for a heterosexual couple.

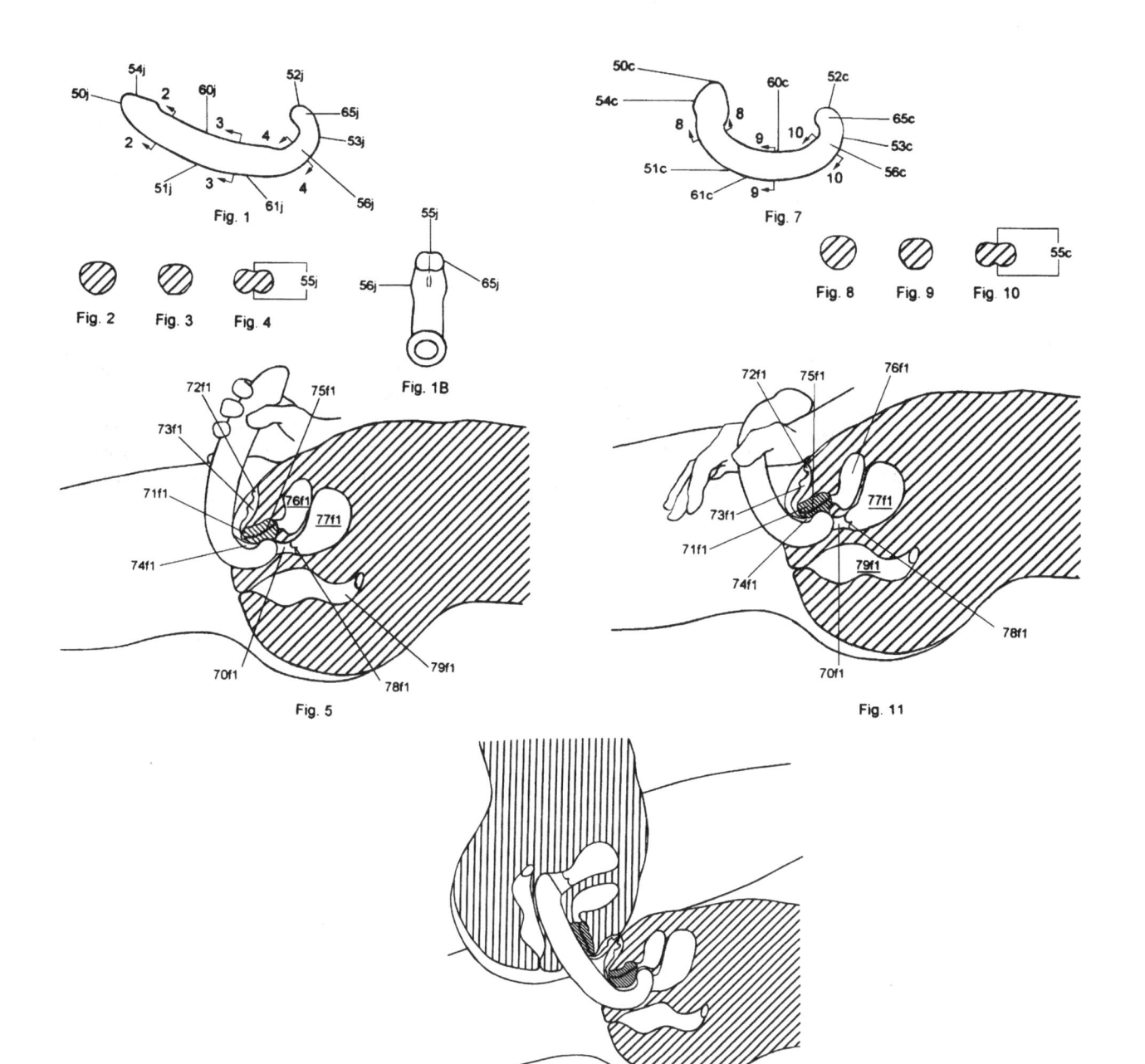

Fig. 1
Fig. 2
Fig. 3
Fig. 4
Fig. 1B
Fig. 5
Fig. 7
Fig. 8
Fig. 9
Fig. 10
Fig. 11
Fig. 6

61

# Hair Circle for Conjugal Affection

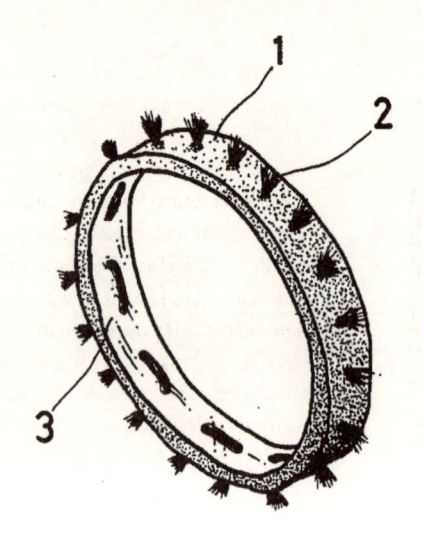

Patent No. 4,854,303
Aug 8, 1989
Dao-Pin Chang

### Abstract

Hair circle for conjugal affection is described. The circle consists of a base member of elastic material having a plurality of mutually spaced round holes extending radially therethrough. A tuft of soft hair extends through each hole with a single tuft extending through a pair of holes. The hair tufts are secured by a adherent film coated on the inner surface of the base member. The tufts may be arranged in rows longitudinally, transverse, or in triangular shapes and the base member can have a cross-section which is rectangular, semicircular, elliptical, or substantially circular.

Patent No. 5,920,923
July 13, 1999
Penn Jillette

# Hydro-Therapeutic Stimulator

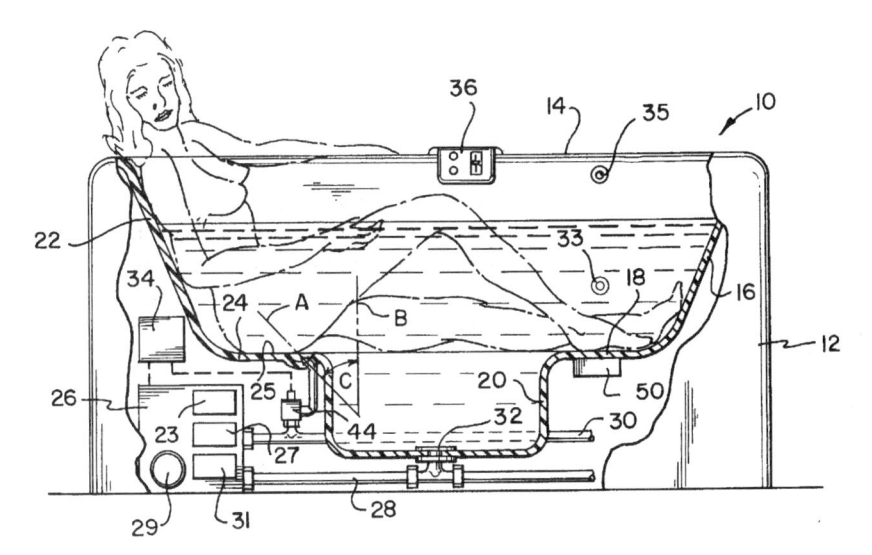

## Abstract

A spa of a type including a tub for holding water and a user, in particular, a female user. The spa has a seat for supporting the female user in a seated position, a circulation pump having an inlet connected to the tub for drawing water from the tub, and an outlet connected to the tub for discharging the drawn water back to the tub. A discharge nozzle is located within the tub and connected to the outlet, mounted to the seat so that the discharged water from the circulation pump automatically aligns with and is directed to stimulation points (e.g., the clitoris) of the female user when the female user sits in the seat.

# Improvement in Uterine Supporters

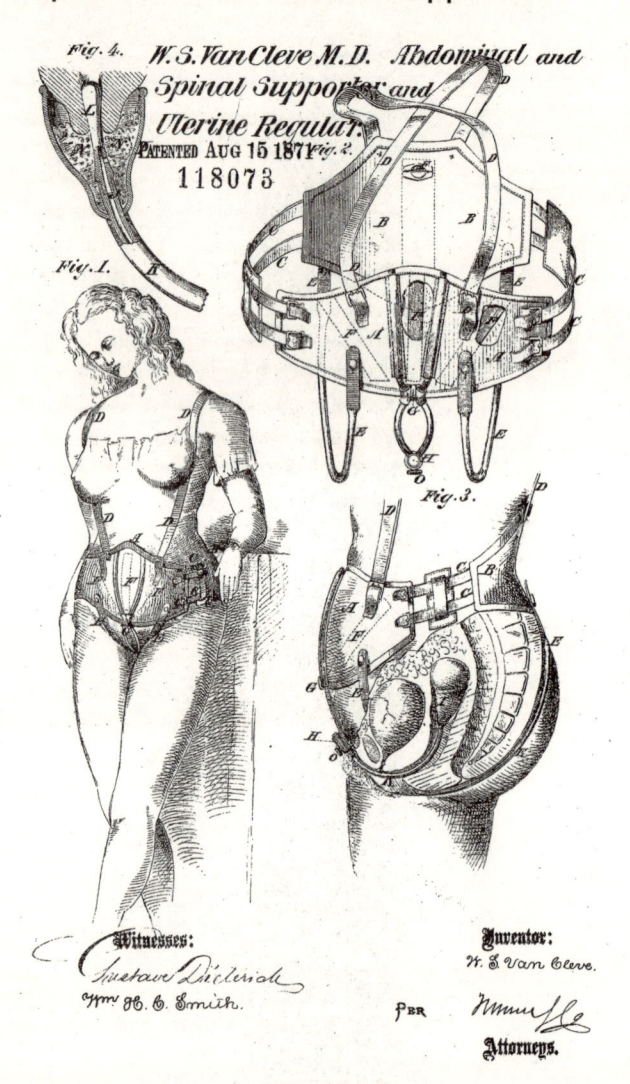

Patent No. 118,073
Aug 15, 1871
William S. Van Cleve

## Abstract

My invention consists in an improvement upon uterine regulators and supporters, as hereinafter fully described and subsequently pointed out in the claim. The figure represents a wide front or abdominal band, and a wide back-band, which are connected together by the adjusting straps and suspended by the shoulder straps. They are also held against rising up by the under straps, passing under and between the thighs.

Patent No. 5,453,080
Sep 26, 1995
John T. Mitchum Jr.

# Intercourse-Facilitating Therapeutic Furniture

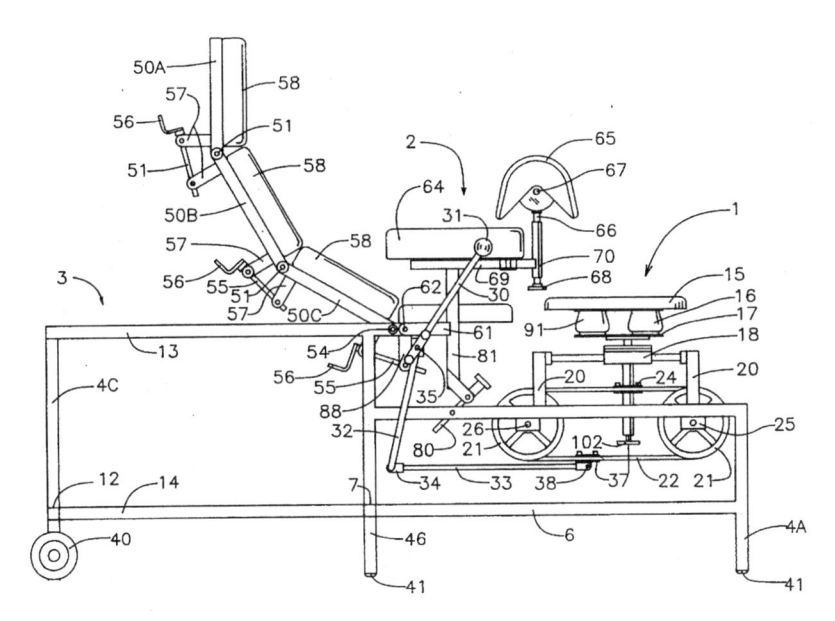

## Abstract

Therapeutic furniture for disabled persons adapted to support man and woman partners engaged in intercourse has longitudinally moveable man's seat facing adjustable-position female seat. Male partner is supported by seat with his back in substantially upright position to relieve stresses on lumbar vertebrae, pelvis and legs. Longitudinal movement of the man's seat is effected by hand operation of a joy stick in mechanical communication with the seat, or, according to a modification of the invention, by actuation of an electric motor in electrical communication with the man's seat. Woman's seat and back are independently adjustable.

Patent No. 6,135,113
Oct 24, 2000
Deloris Gray Wood

# Kissing Shield and Method of Use Thereof

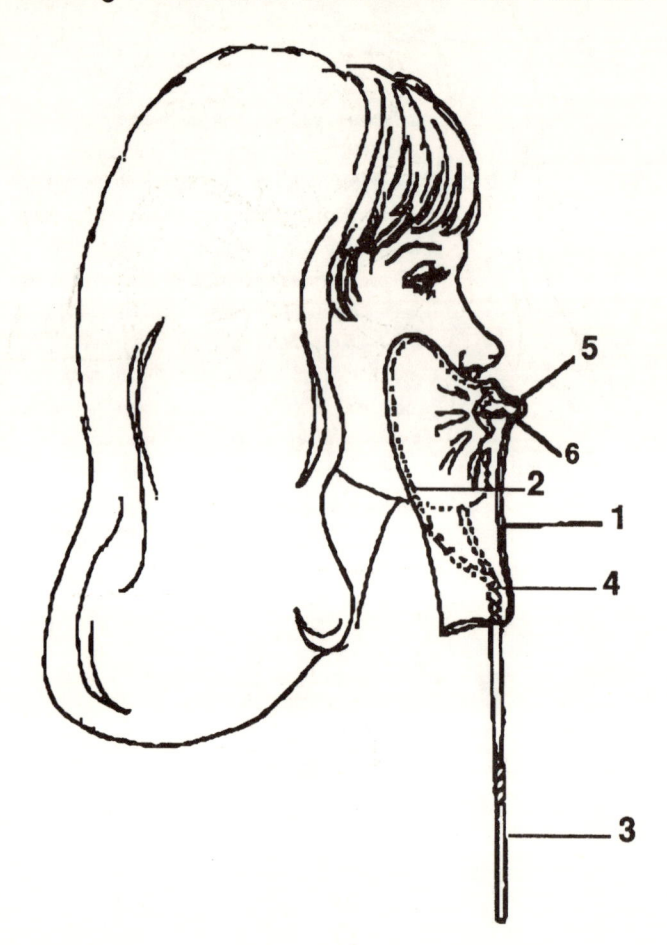

## Abstract

A kissing shield is comprised of a thin, flexible membrane and a frame or holder. The membrane is closed on three sides, a fourth side remaining open so that the membrane can be stretched over the frame or holder. The frame or holder consists of a supporting member and an elongated handle. The supporting member adapts over the bottom part of the user's face and has sufficient dimension to cover the lips and most of the cheeks and extends from under the nose to the bottom of the chin. The elongated handle extends laterally from the supporting member and is sized to be held in the hand of the user such that the hand is spaced apart from the supporting member and membrane. In use, the membrane is placed over the frame or holder. Using the handle portion of the frame or holder, the user places the kissing shield under his nose, so that it covers his lips, cheeks and chin. The user then positions the kissing shield between his lips and the lips or cheek of the individual he plans to kiss and kisses the intended recipient of his affection.

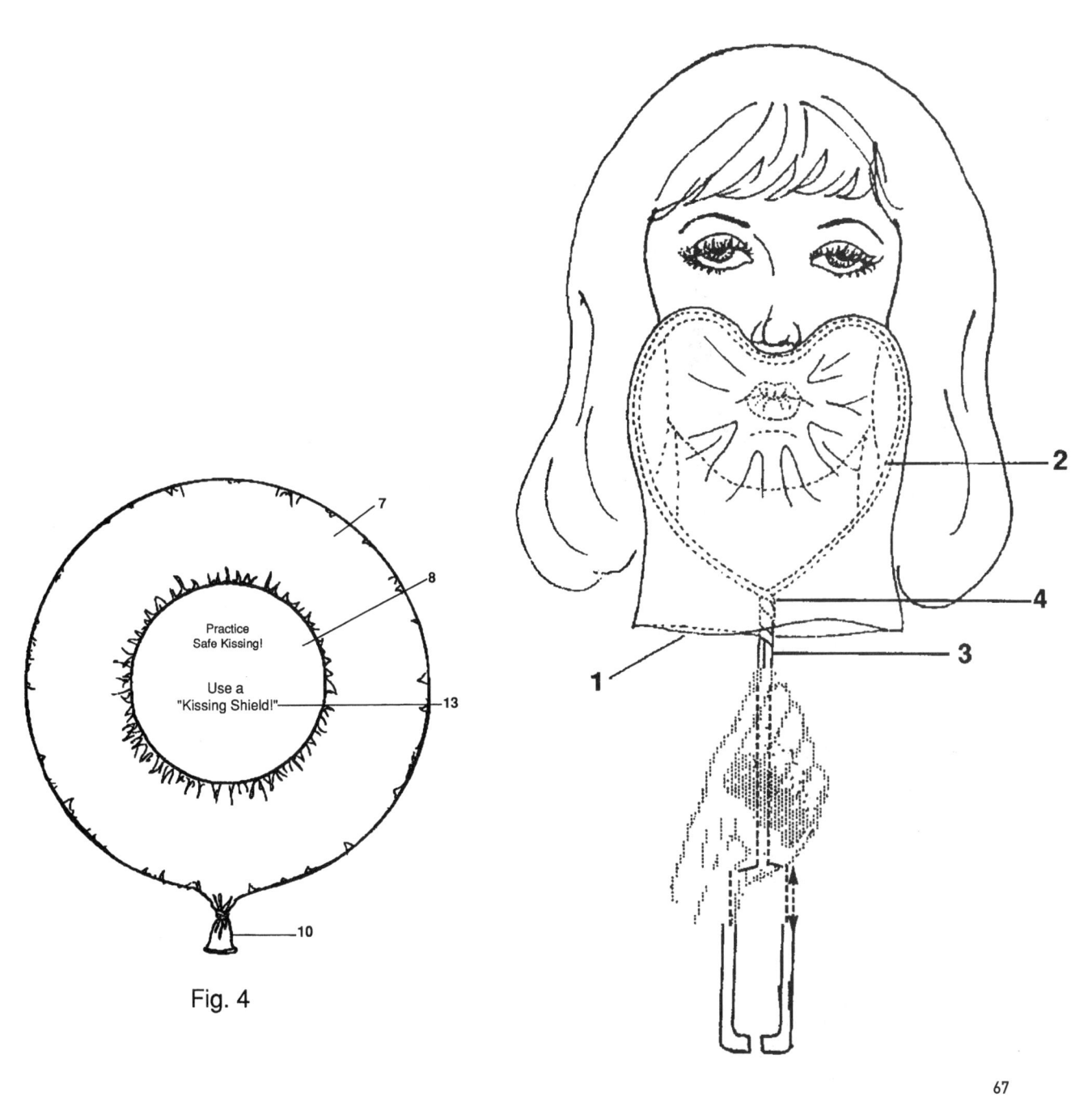

Fig. 4

# Lap Dance Liner

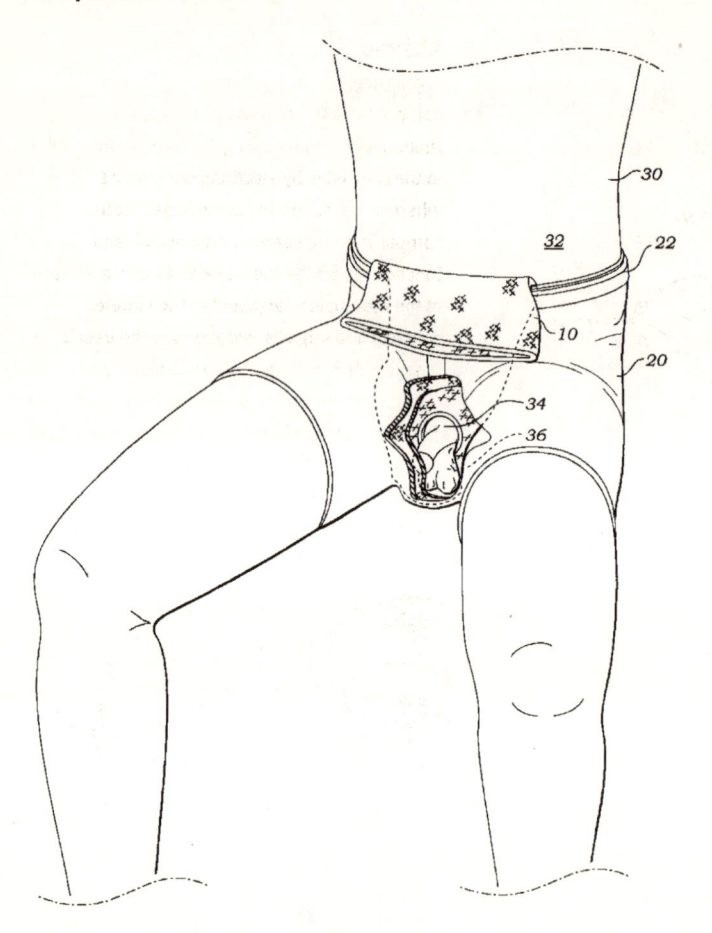

Patent No. US 6,406,462 B1
Jun 18, 2002
Wesley Johnson

## Abstract

A combination pouch and underwear pant is worn by a man for facilitating sexual activity such as lap dancing. The pouch is worn over the sex organs of a man under the underwear pant, which is adapted by an elastic waistband for compressively pinning the pouch in place. The pouch is made of a flexible and elastic material. A top edge of the pouch provides access to an interior of the pouch of a hand and wrist of the wearer so as to facilitate insertion of the wearer's sex organs into the pouch through an aperture, which encircles penis and scrotum. The aperture elastically compresses between a top surface at the base of the penis of the wearer and a bottom surface at the base of the scrotum of the wearer. With the pouch in place, the wearer is able to facilitate the capture of body fluids without fear of the pouch moving away from its preferred position relative to the torso of the wearer.

Patent No. US 6,645,164 B2
Nov 11, 2003
Wayne E. Manska

# Lingual Vibration Device

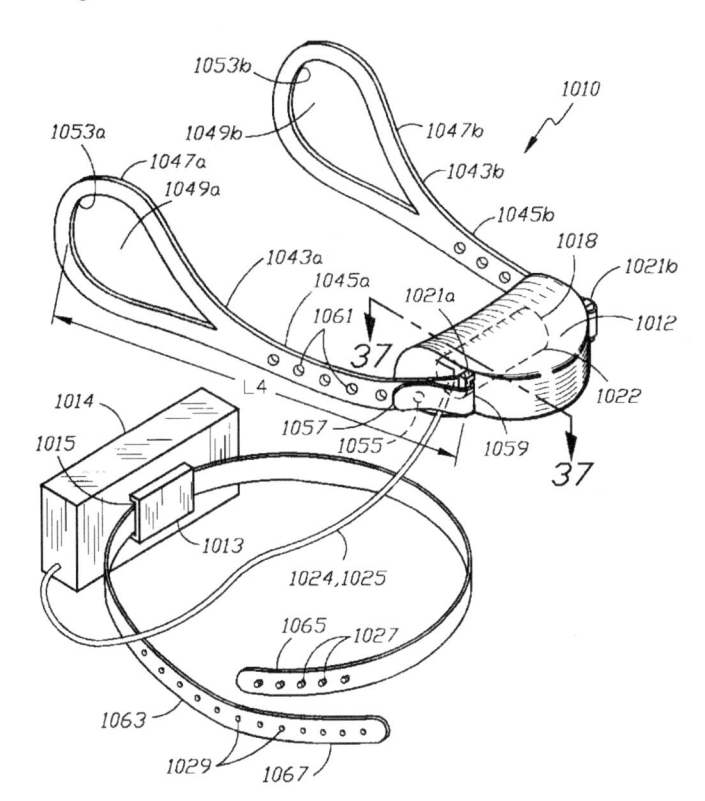

## Abstract

A vibrating oral sex enhancement device comprising a mouthpiece and a controller. The mouthpiece retains a vibrator that is connected to the controller by electrical conductors, whereas the controller comprises a battery compartment, a battery and a switch and functions to power the vibrator. In use, a surface of the mouthpiece adjacent to the vibrator contacts and imparts vibrations to the user's tongue, which results in increased sexual pleasure to the user's partner during oral sex. The device is comfortably stabilized in the user's mouth such that vibrations are optimally imparted to the tongue while leaving the tongue free to move with respect to the mouthpiece.

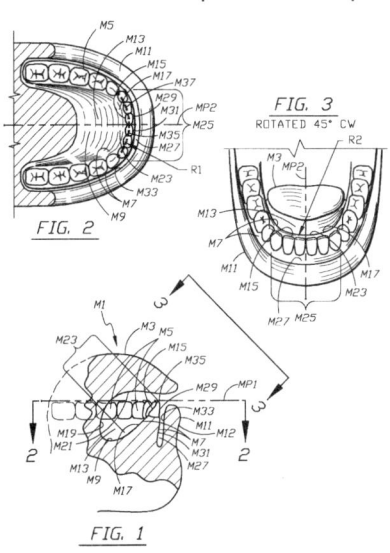

Patent No. 5,213,509
May 25, 1993
John C. Gunn

# Lover's Game and Method of Play

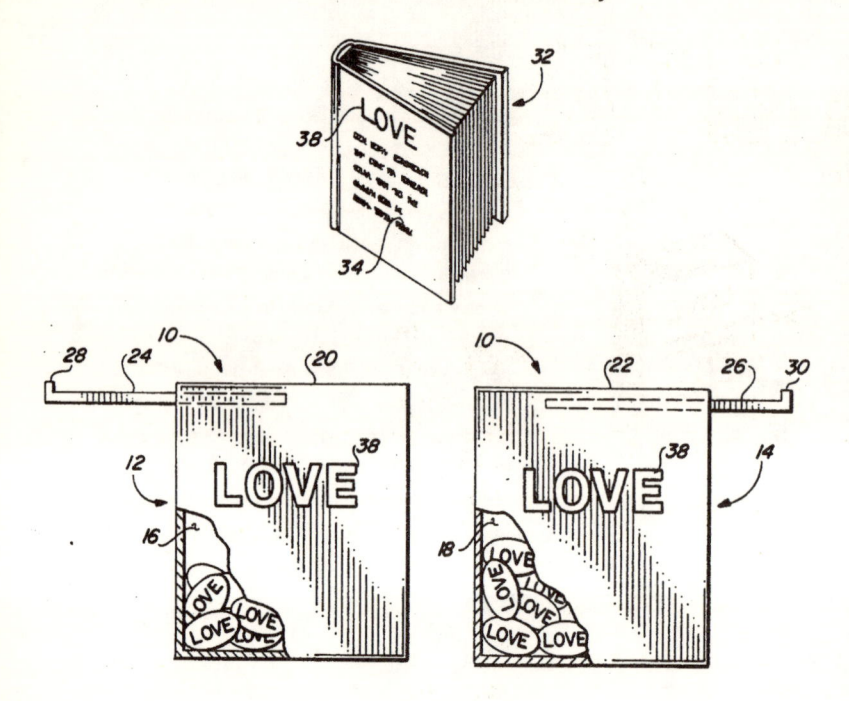

## Abstract

The game for lovers includes two open-topped containers, with or without closeable top lids and central storage spaces, and a number of game pieces of sufficiently small size so that a number of the pieces can fit into each space. The total number of pieces in the game is more than enough to fill one of the spaces, but insufficient to fill both spaces. Most preferably, they are in the form of different simulated jewels of various sizes, shapes and appearances. In one embodiment, the rules guide, containers and/or pieces bear the legend "lovers". Whenever a lover performs a loving act, he or she gives the other lover a game piece which is stored in the recipient's container space. When the pieces overflow a container that is the signal for the lover having that container to perform a sufficient number of loving acts and distribute the overflowing pieces to the other participant thus promoting harmony and exchanging and sharing of loving acts between the game lovers.

Fig-1b

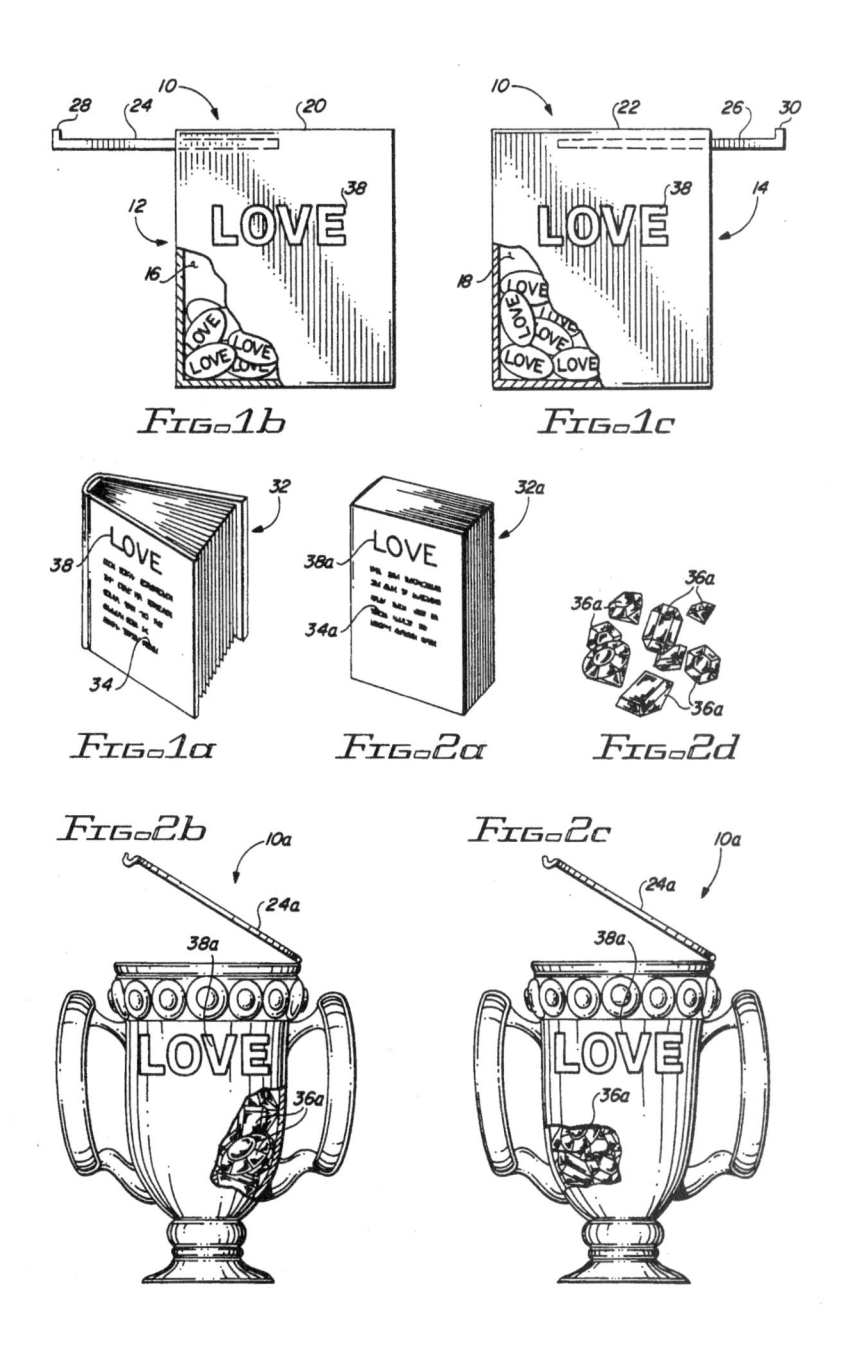

Fig-1c

Fig-1a

Fig-2a

Fig-2d

Fig-2b

Fig-2c

Patent No. 5,237,706
Aug 24, 1993
Robert M. Nalbandian

# Male Garment with Scrotal Pouch

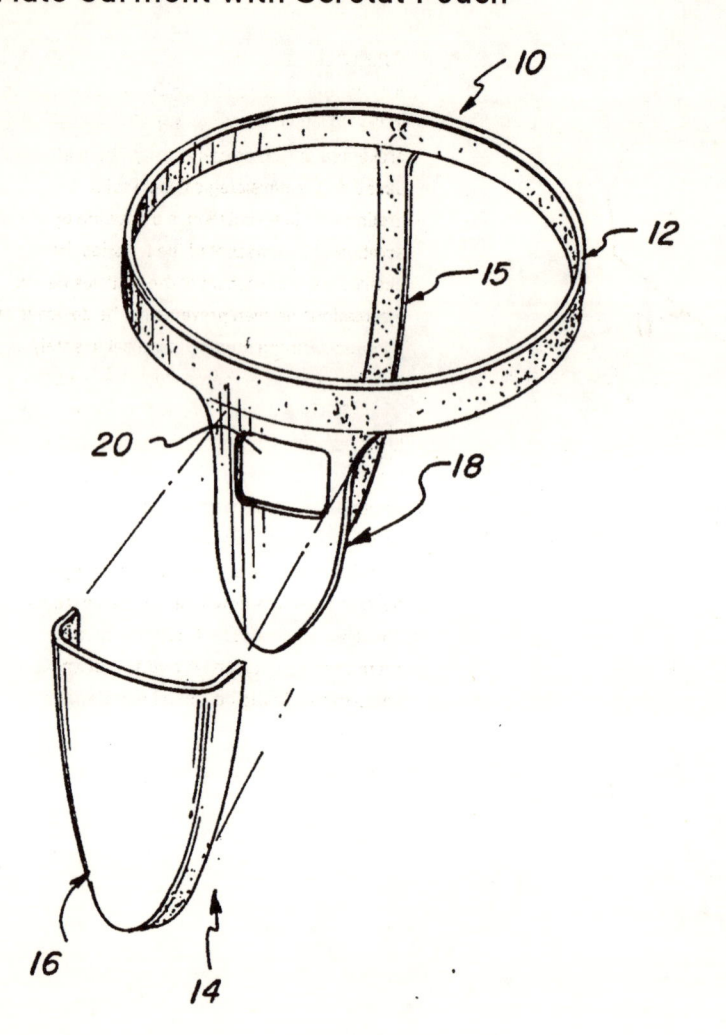

### Abstract

The present invention provides a male garment with a scrotal pouch. More specifically, the present invention provides a male garment with a scrotal pouch comprising an anterior panel and a posterior panel with an opening in said posterior panel to enable the continuous anterior displacement of the penis and scrotum in the usual anatomic relationship to one another.

Patent No. 5,063,915
Nov 12, 1991
Robert L. Wyckoff

# Male Genital Device and Method for Control of Ejaculation

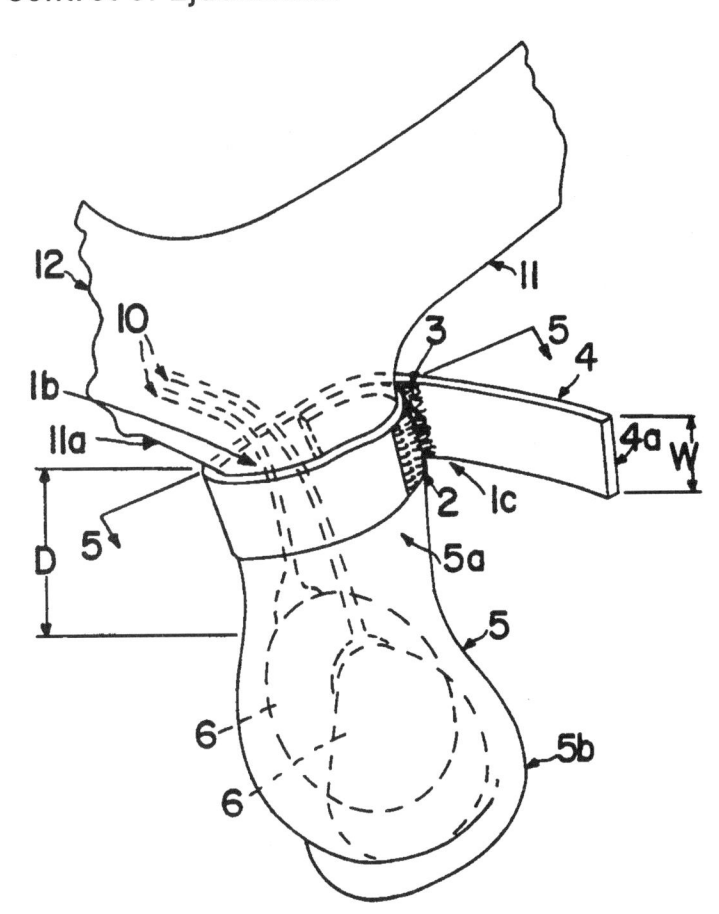

## Abstract

A method and device by which sexual emission in the male can be delayed or alternatively prevented during sexual activity. The method is based on the physiological fact that a preliminary to ejaculation is a drawing up of the scrotum and an ascent of the testicles. Hence, obstructing such ascent of the testicles delays ejaculations or even prevents it. The device is an annulus-forming member applicable solely around the neck of the scrotum, the annulus formed being of a size barring passage of the testicles so as to obstruct their ascent. The member does not cause pain or discomfort, and does not encumber sexual activity. Further, the annulus formed is easily released and the member removed entirely, if desired, by either party to influence timing of ejaculation readily. The device is useful for treatment of male premature ejaculation as well as treatment, in some cases, of frigidity in the female.

# Male Genital Strengthening Device

Patent No. D258,690
Mar 24, 1981
An C. Wu

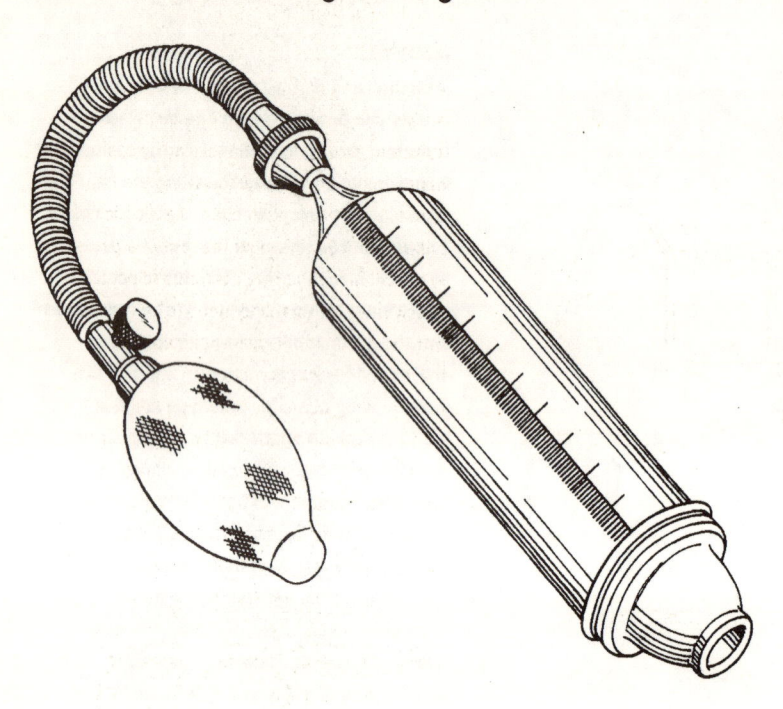

## Abstract
The figure is a perspective view of a male genital strengthening device showing my new design, the undisclosed side being the mirror image thereof less the graduations.

Patent No. 4,539,980
Sep 10, 1985
John L. Chaney

# Male Organ Conditioner

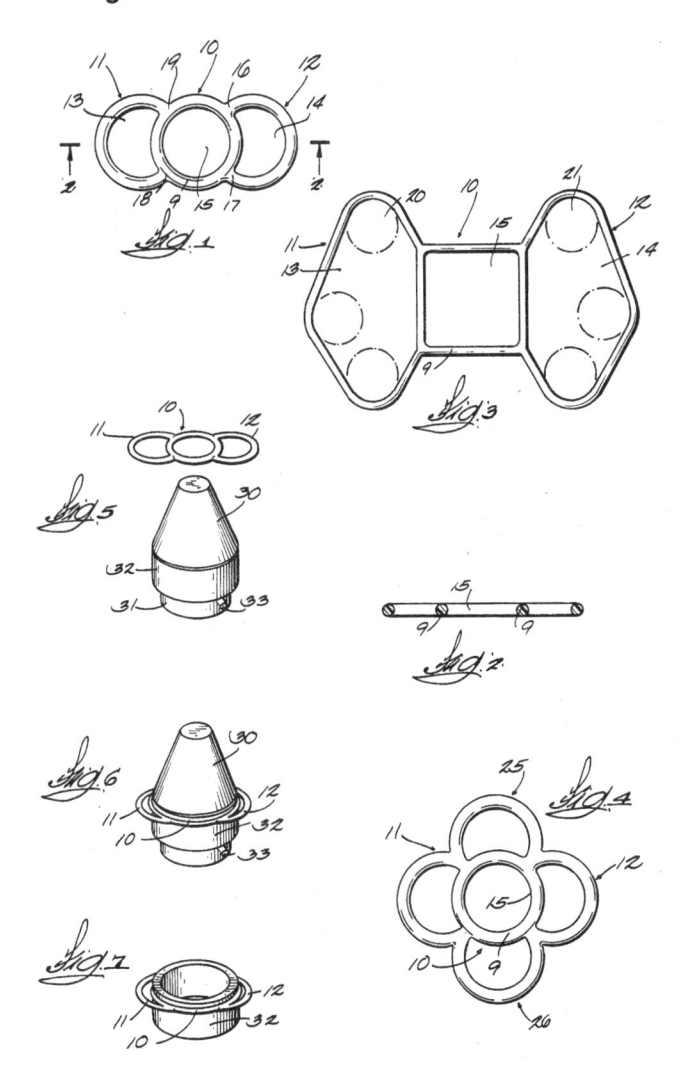

## Abstract

A central elastic ring having elastic loops attached to opposite sides. The loops are of sufficient size to insert fingers on opposite hands into them whereupon when the hands are spread away from each other the elastic ring enlarges for being set on the root of a penis. When released the ring contracts to act as a check valve for enabling blood to be massaged into the penis and to prevent its outflow to thereby obtain and maintain an erection. An accessory provides for mounting the elastic ring on a rigid sleeve which can be fitted over the penis so the elastic ring can be slid off at the root of the penis.

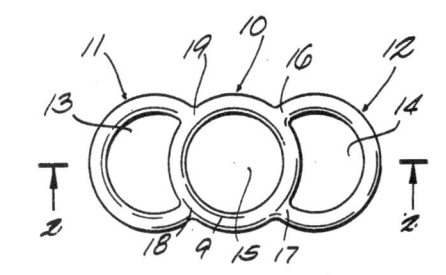

Patent No. US 4,640,270
Feb 3, 1987
Te-Chien Chin

# Male Organ Jacket

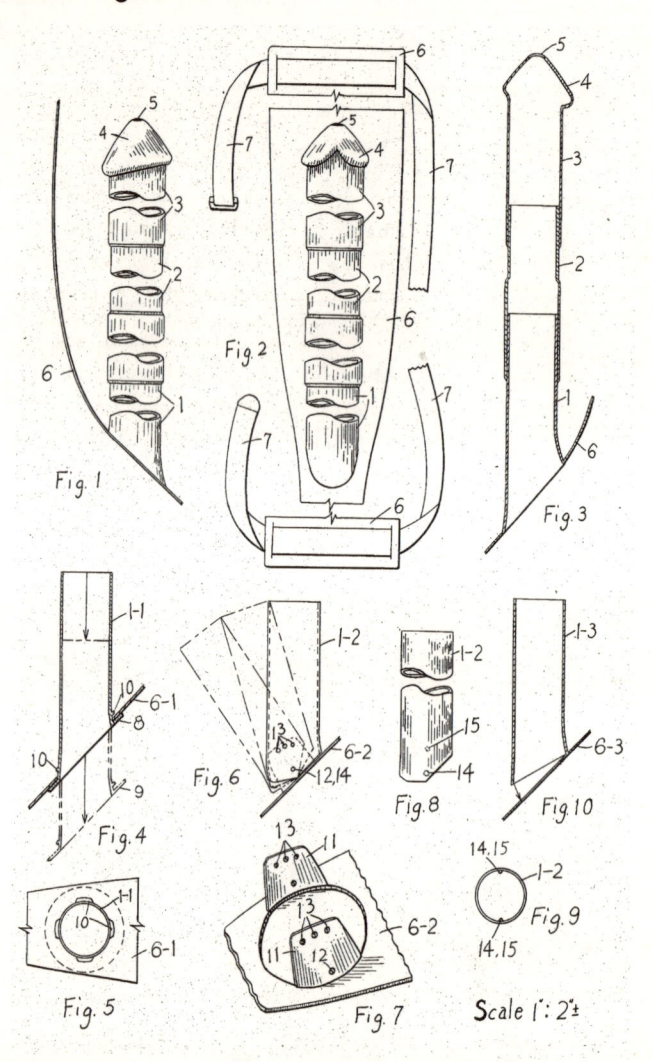

## Abstract

Disclosed is a sex aid device for supporting and/or strengthening the penis, especially the imperfect ones, comprising a semi-rigid three-sectioned casing of adjustable length. The sections of the casing are optional except the base section. A supporting strap with various connecting means connects the casing to the male body at different angles.

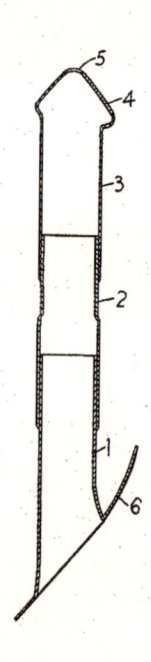

Patent No. 4,672,954
June 16, 1987
Jack S. Panzer

# Male Sexual Aid Holder

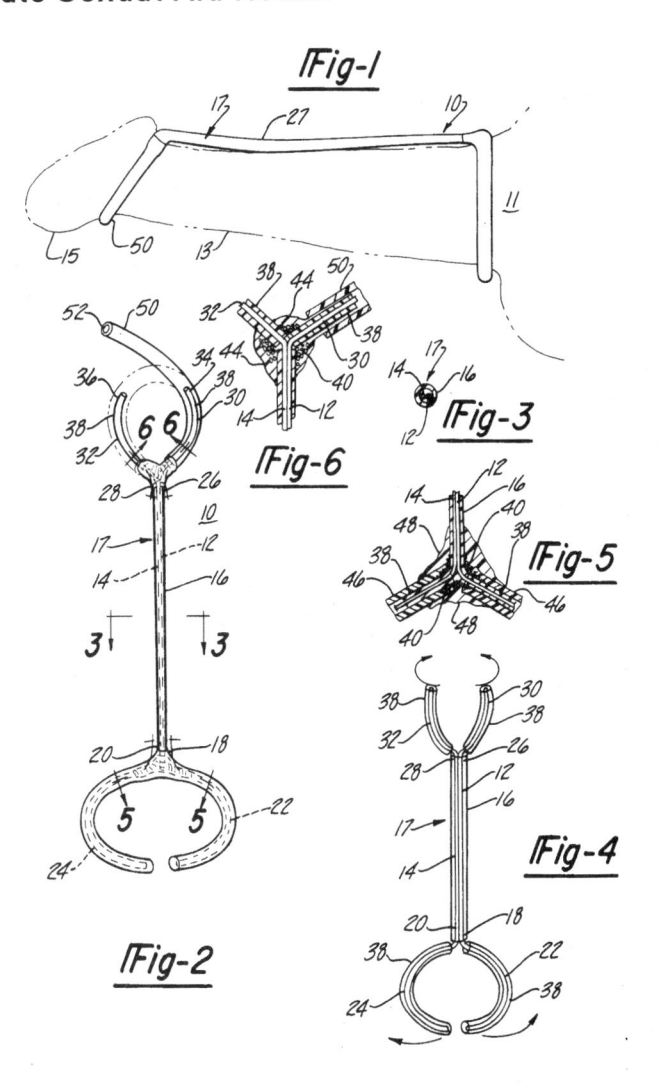

## Abstract

A genital splint for permitting a human male to achieve penetration during sexual intercourse is easily sized to individual penile diameters, yet is both positively secured and readily removable from the penis. Pairs of arcuate members are affixed to the ends of the rod so as to form a base ring closely fitting about the root of the penis, and a collar closely fitting about the corona of the penis.

Patent No. 1,210,809
Jan 2, 1917
Johannes Christian Johansen

# Massage Apparatus

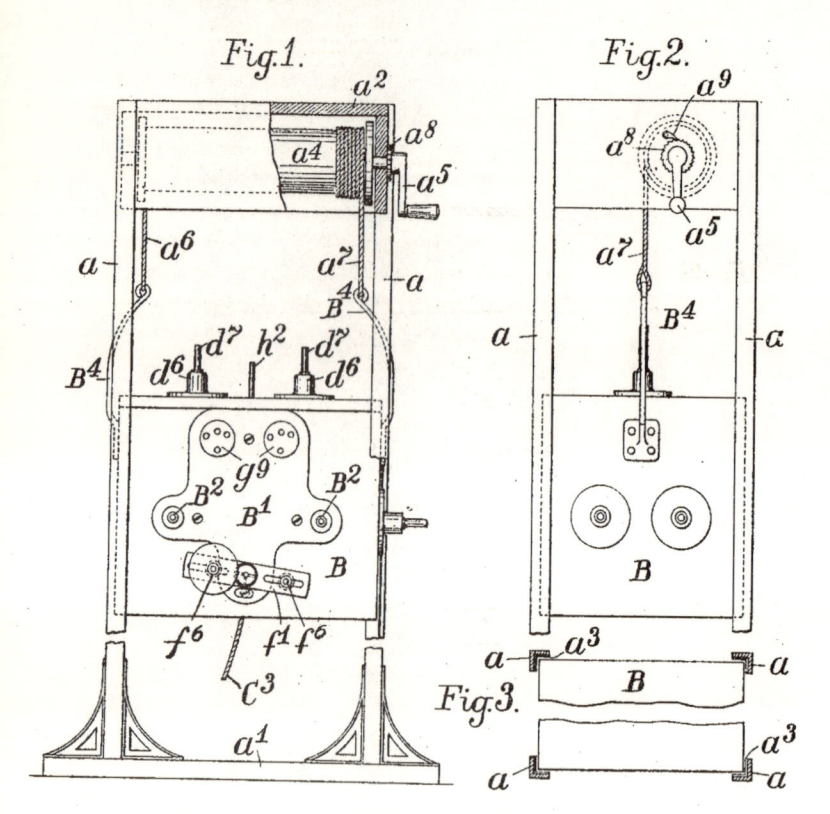

## Abstract

The present invention relates to massage apparatus of the stationary type in contradiction to those apparatus which are held in the hand, and although usually the apparatus will be used in a certain position, it is preferably made so that it can be adjusted, moved or even inclined or turned on one of its sides. The object of the invention is to provide an apparatus which shall be capable of use under all conditions and for all purposes for which the massage apparatus may be required and to so construct the machine that while it is provided with a number of tools or applicators, or means for applying a number of tools or applicators in different positions, the mechanism is provided in a comparatively small compass and is sufficiently protected against damage or interference while it is preferably so mounted or arranged so as to be capable of being adjusted both vertically (or horizontally) and angularly.

Fig. 14.  Fig. 15.  Fig. 16.

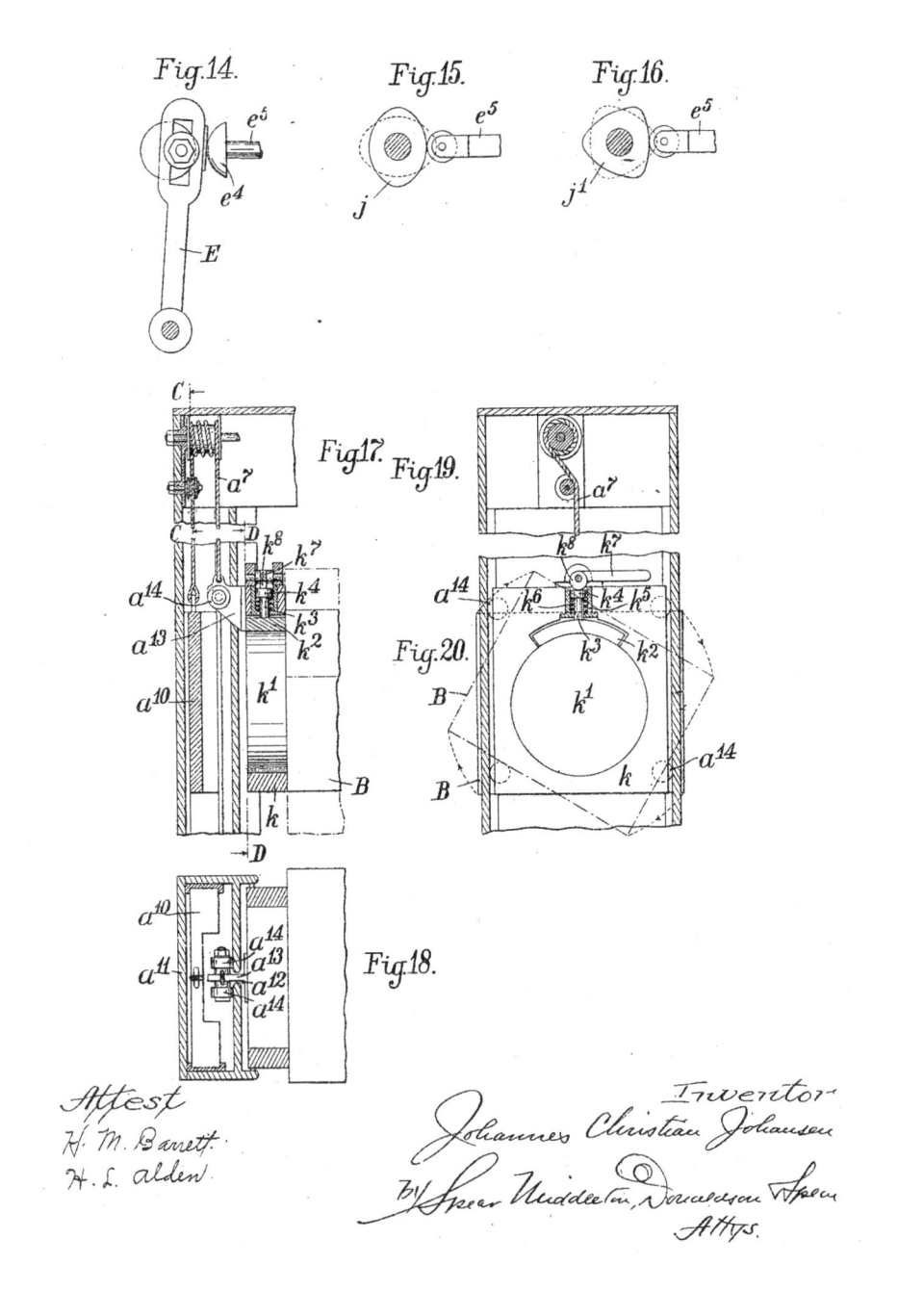

Fig. 17.  Fig. 19.

Fig. 20.

Fig. 18.

Attest
H. M. Barrett.
H. L. Alden.

Inventor
Johannes Christian Johansen
By Spear Middleton, Donaldson Spear
Attys.

# Massage Device

Patent No. 5,470,303
Nov 28, 1995
Cynthia D. Leonard; Lawrence Gayne

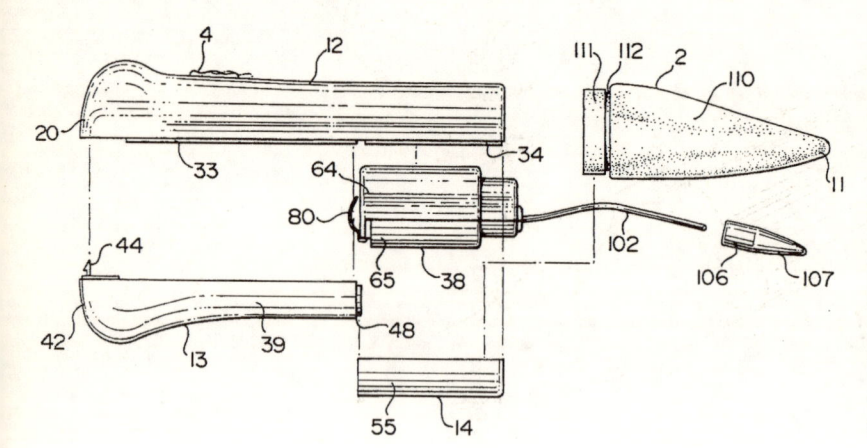

## Abstract

Conventional massage devices of the sexual self-stimulator type include reciprocating massage heads. Some devices of this type feature rotary massage heads. A novel device includes a housing containing a drive and carrying a soft, flexible, resilient, tongue-shaped head on one end thereof, the head containing an arcuate shaft with a straight inner end connected to the drive, whereby the path of travel of the shaft during rotation defines an ellipsoid with a cone on the outer free end thereof.

FIG. 1

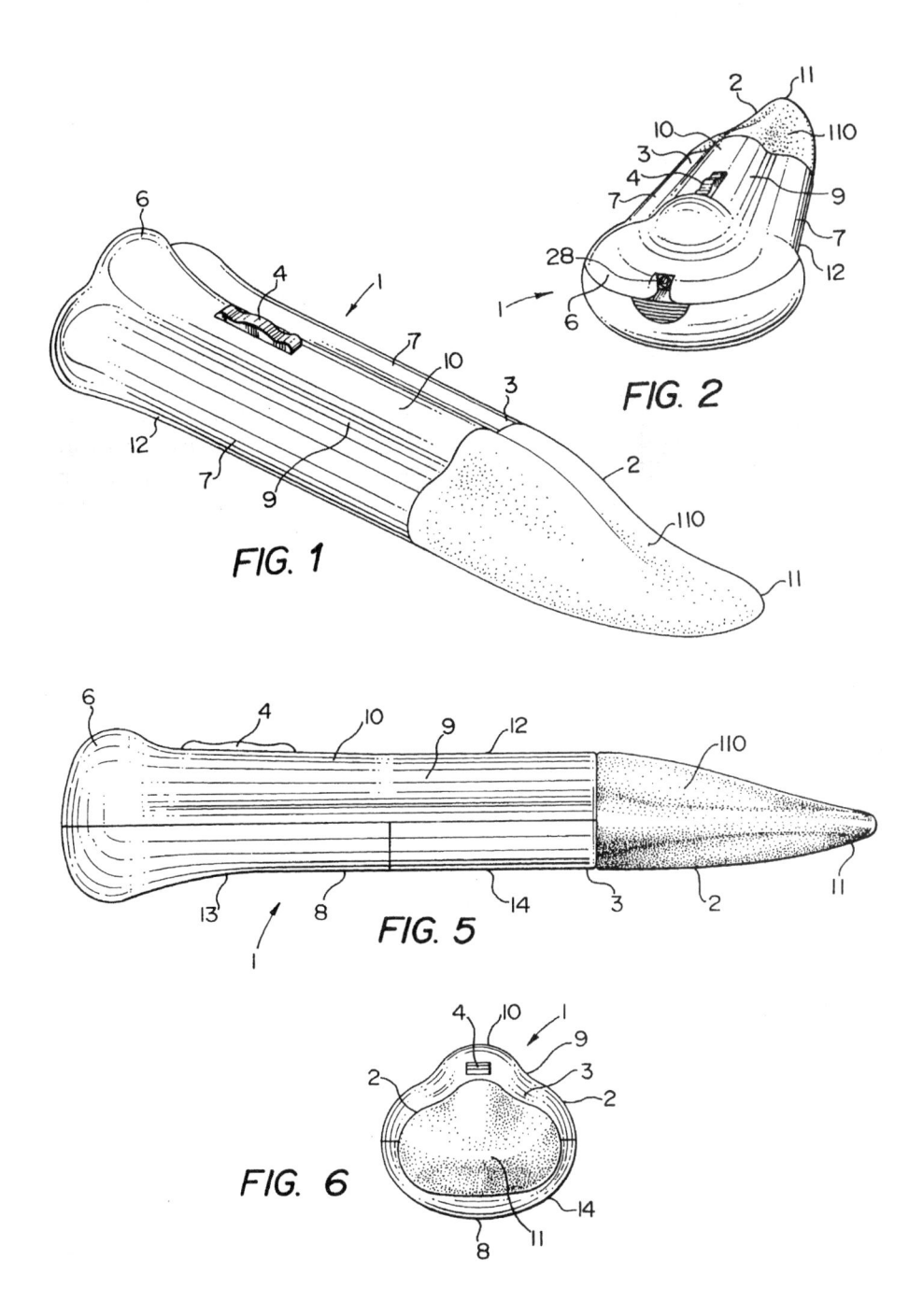

FIG. 2

FIG. 5

FIG. 6

# Massaging Apparatus for Penis

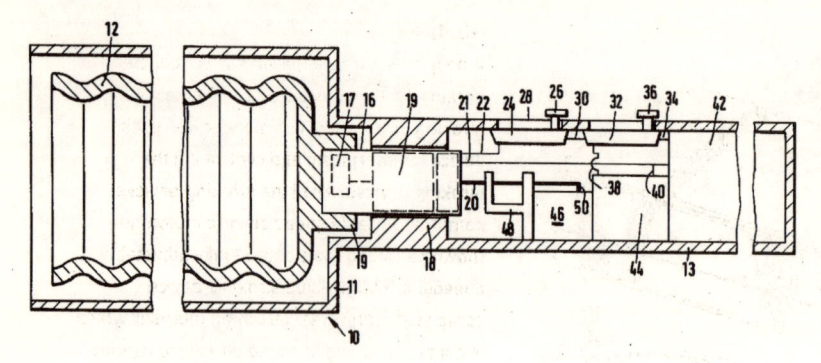

Patent No. 4,059,100
Nov 22, 1977
Ulrich Glage

## Abstract

An apparatus for massaging elongated parts of the human body, especially for applying massage to stimulate and improve the ability for erection, comprises an elongated sheath which is excitable to controlled vibrations of two superimposed frequencies.

Patent No. 3,978,851
Sep 7, 1976
P. Brav Sobel

# Massaging Apparatus (with Stroking Device)

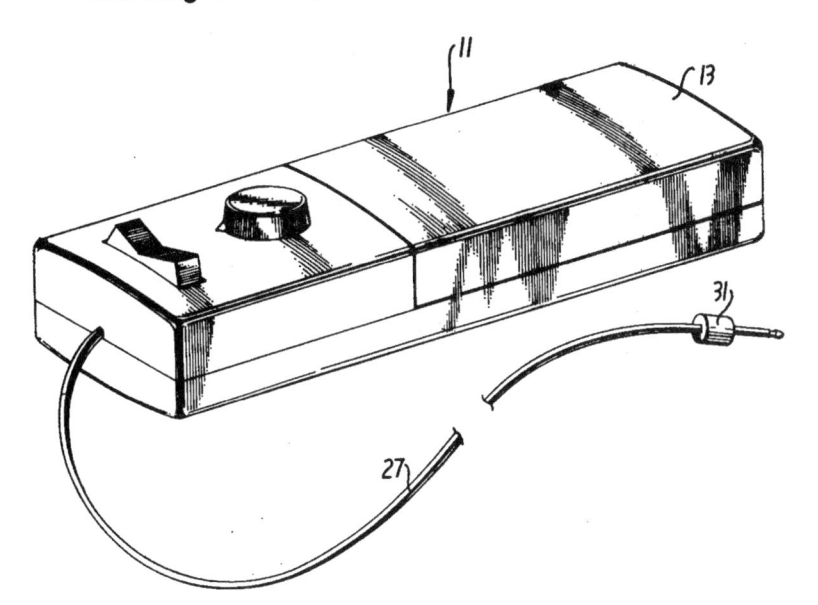

## Abstract

A body massaging apparatus is described herein which includes a plurality of separate stroking devices and a remote power-pack device for energizing and controlling the stroking devices. All of the stroking devices comprise variable speed electric motors for moving stroking tools at gradually adjustable speeds. A rotating-type stroking-device comprises a universal attaching member which is capable of being attached directly to various types of limp, flexible, stroking materials for rotating them. A clasping-type stroking device comprises a housing with an elongated jaw member pivotally attached to the housing. A gripping-type stroking device comprises a housing with two gripping members, each having at least two gripping arms, extending outwardly from the housing. A rotational/swinging stroking device comprises a cylindrical helical-spring stroking tool which can be both rotated along a longitudinal axis or pivoted in a swinging motion.

Patent No. 6,061,840
May 16, 2000
Squire Alligator

# Men's Anatomic Underwear/Swimwear

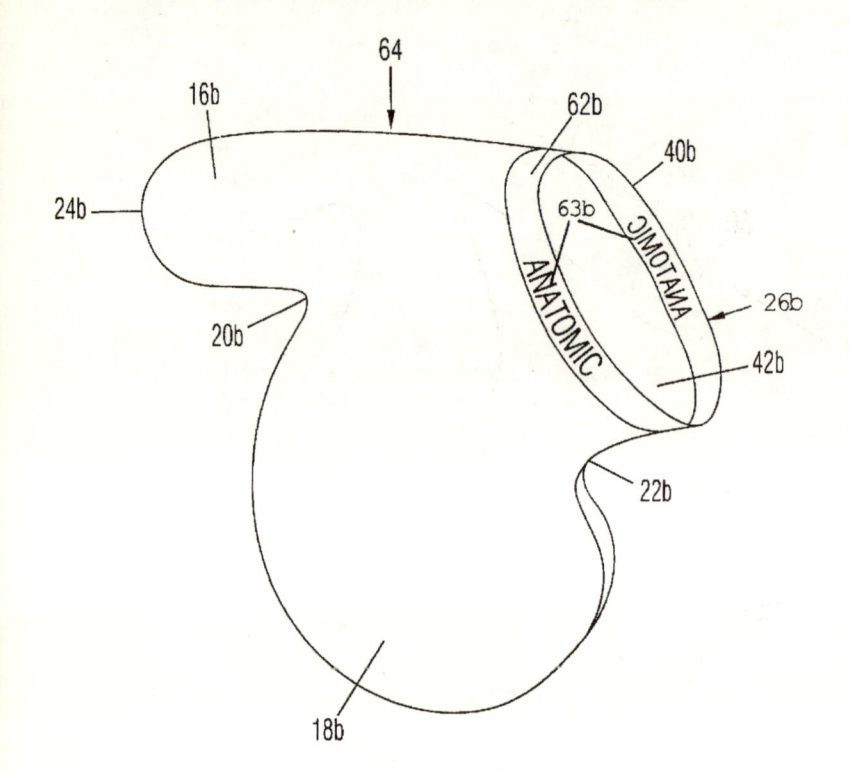

## Abstract

A male brief, specifically underwear, swimwear, sunwear, supporter, medical brief, or enhancement device is designed to be worn instead of men's usual underwear and swimwear. The brief's form follows the anatomical design of the penis and the scrotum, which are two naturally separated, yet integrated entities. To achieve superior support and comfort the brief is designed to accurately conform to the changing shapes, movements and precise positions that the genitals make of their own accord to maintain comfort and health. This allows the genitals to dictate their own comfort, and at the same time be held by the brief in a protective and supportive way. Because the brief is configured to reflect the exact contours of the genitals, it possesses unadulterated lines that house the genitals with a never-before-achieved attractiveness by allowing their natural carriage and authentic masculine style to be expressed in a way that reflects their own image. A fly system built into pouch allows for the release of the penis for urinating without having to remove the brief.

Fig. 1c

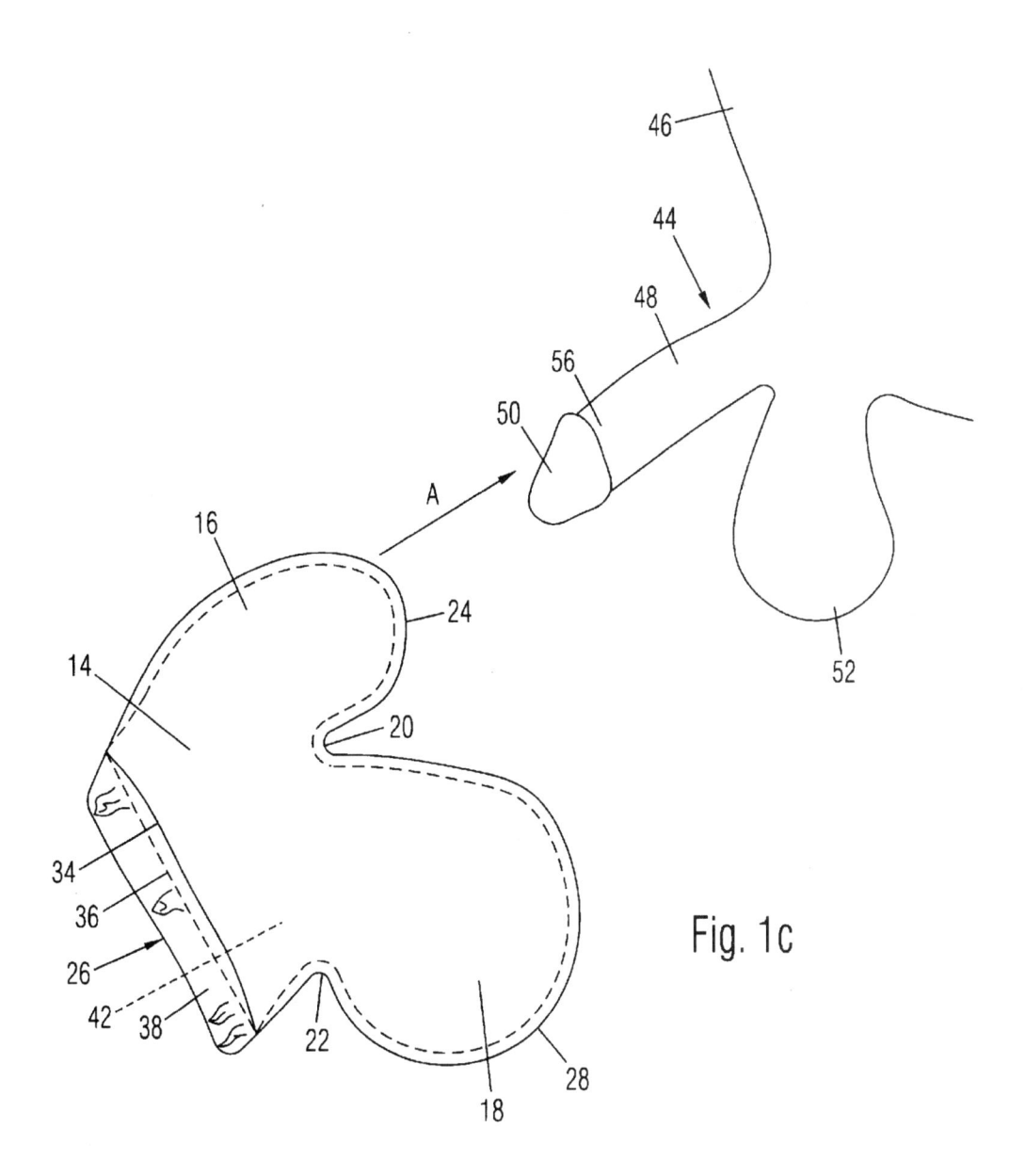

Patent No. 5,239,841
Aug 31, 1993
Hans Zwart

# Method for Decorating a Human Breast

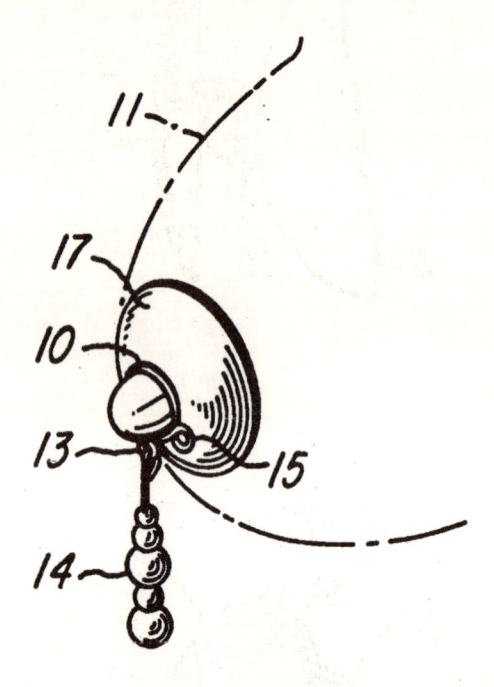

## Abstract

A spring wire or other spring-like material is formed with a circular ring portion which has a diameter adapted to fit snugly around a nipple of a human breast. The wire or material also forms two overlapping end portions which project outwardly from the ring portion and are compressed together to enlarge the ring portion so that it may be conveniently placed on the nipple and removed from the nipple. When the end portions are released, the ring portion grips the peripheral surface of the nipple. Preferably, the end portions comprise smaller circular rings which may be used to support different forms of jewelry, and the ring portion may also support a decorative element which covers the nipple. The ring portion and end portions are decorated, preferably by plating with a precious metal.

FIG-7

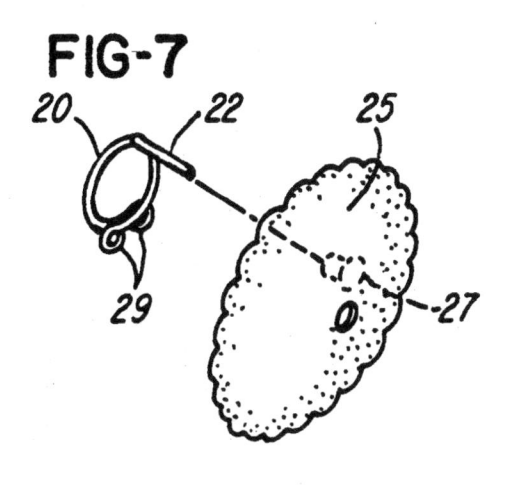

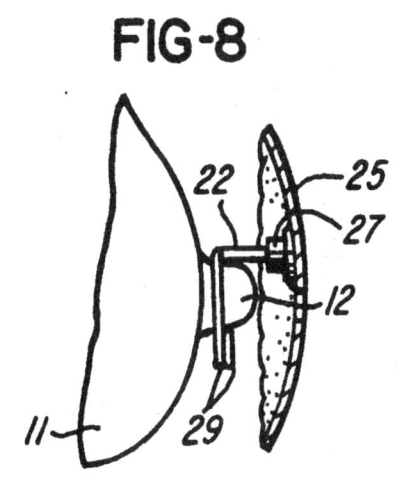

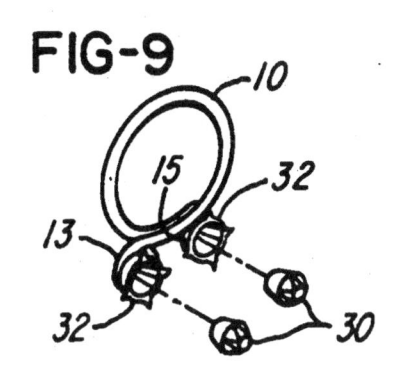

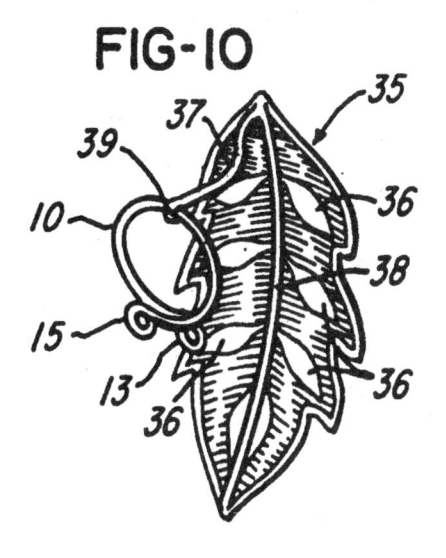

FIG-8

FIG-9

FIG-10

# Method of Inducing Safety in Sexual Acts and Aids in Support Thereof

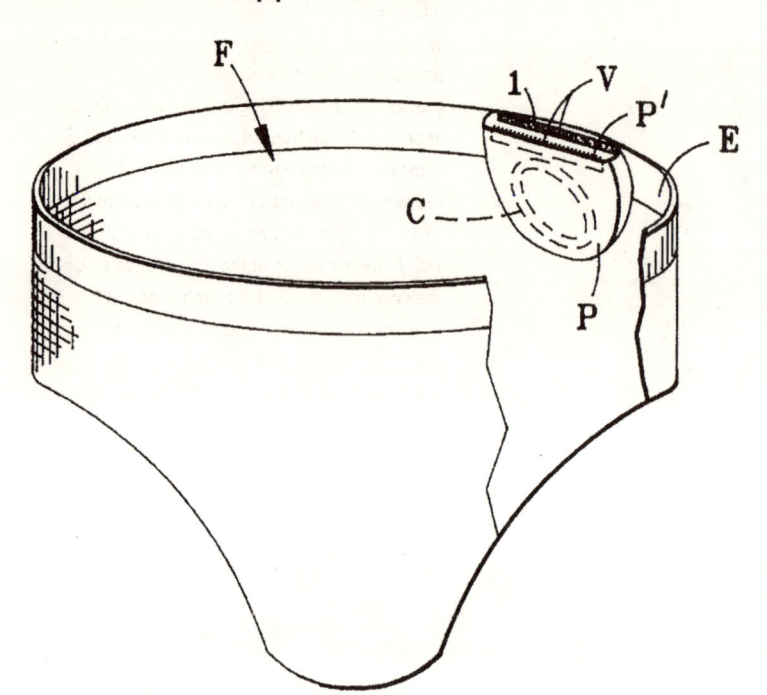

Patent No. 5,460,188
Oct 24, 1995
Ronald A. Barrett Sr.

## Abstract

A method and garment aid to facilitate and induce the use of a condom for safe or safer sexual acts are disclosed, wherein a pocket containing a condom is carried, for example, at the inner forward waistband region of the underpants, such that a potential participant, when removing such underpants, as a general precondition to engaging in the sexual act, will invariably touch or be conscious of the pocket-and-condom, thus providing a warning and a reminder of the proximal presence and readily accessible convenience of the juxtaposed condom that may serve to induce use of the same and thereby increase the chances of the enactment of safe or safer sex. Novel pockets including modified condom-package-pockets are disclosed.

Patent No. 5,842,969
Dec 1, 1998
Gennady Alexeevich Vikhrev

# Method of Sexual Disharmony Correction During the Sexual Act

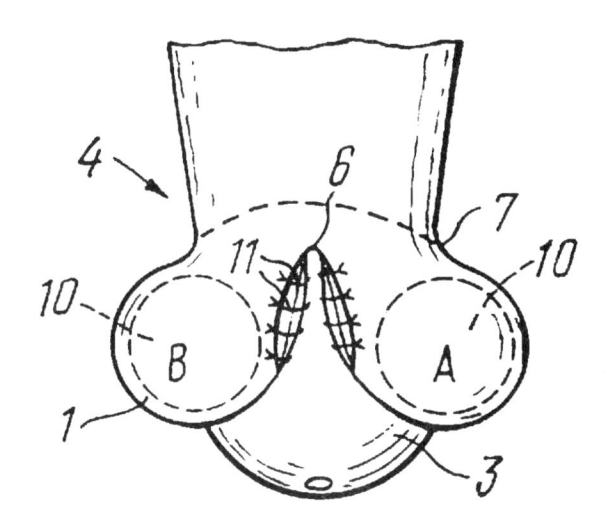

## Abstract

The method of correction of sexual disharmony brings about the stimulation of feminine erogenous zones during the sexual act by way of an aimed mechanical action on the area of clitoris and of the vagina of ball-like elements made from biologically inert materials of 8 to 15 mm in diameter implanted in a numbers of 1 or 2 into the edges of the slit prepuce or under the skin of the penis in a number of 1 to 3 of 5 to 10 mm in diameter and also by the ends of a diameter fixed to the frenulum of the prepuce by 4 to 5 knots through it of 1 to 1.5 mm in diameter.

Patent No. 5,592,144
Jan 7, 1997
James W. Greene

# Mood Lamp

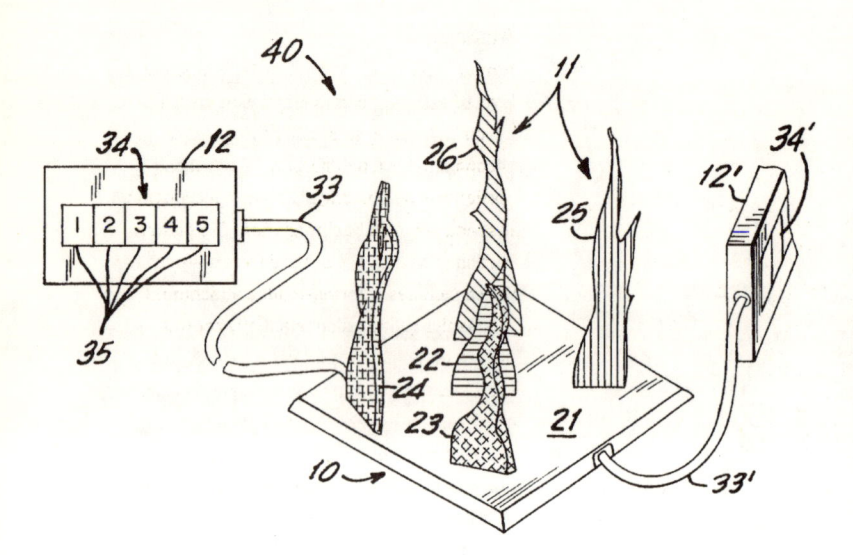

## Abstract

A lamp device for communicating moods between users having a base with a plurality of individually illuminatable elements extending from the base and two control units remote from the base for regulating the illumination of the elements. In a preferred embodiment, the illuminatable elements are in the form of five translucent flames of various heights containing two small electric bulbs at their bases for selectively producing colored illumination of each. Two persons involved in using the lamp for communication each operate a respective control unit which may be concealed, if desired, and by which a level of illumination may be selected to indicate, for instance, the level of interest of the user. When the user couple fails to synchronize their "levels", there is no illumination, but upon synchronization, a flame of an appropriate color will light up. Each level may be assigned specific understood psychological definitions that identify the mood or attitude of the users.

Patent No. US 6,547,717 B1
Apr 15, 2003
John P. Green; Jeffery Sigler

# Multifacet Sexual Aid

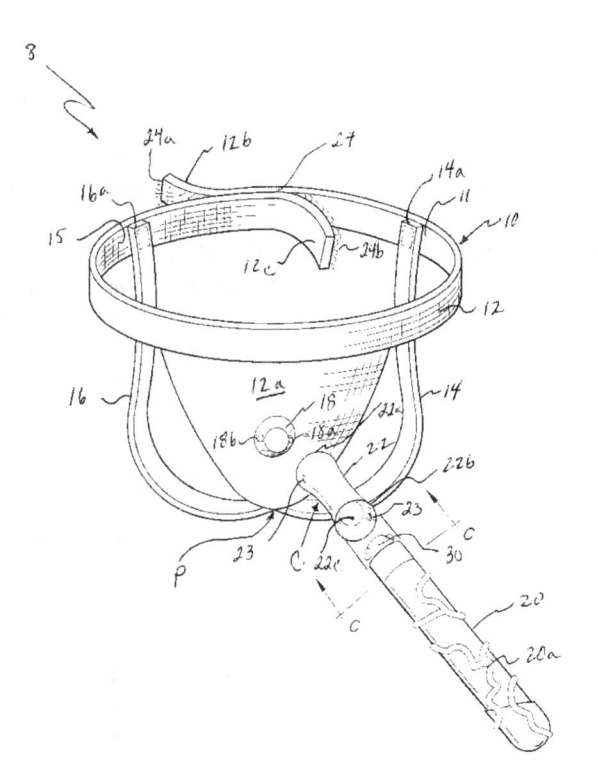

## Abstract

A multifacet sexual aid device for increasing the level of sexual enjoyment between partners which includes a waist belt having a first, second and third belt portion. The first belt portion has a substantially planar portion and a first and second attachment end. The planar portion is a parabolic shaped front element which includes a spring-loaded attachment mechanism within a substantially central portion of the planar portion for attaching at least one prosthetic phallic element thereto, as a quick release and quickly deployed element. A couple connector is also used to couple a plurality of different prosthetic phallic elements as either a convex or concave connection to the spring-loaded mechanism. The free ends of each second and third belt portions are fixedly secured at opposing internal first and second internal surface portions via hook and loop fasteners.

Patent No. 5,782,672
July 21, 1998
Vickie G. Woodley

# Nipple Pad

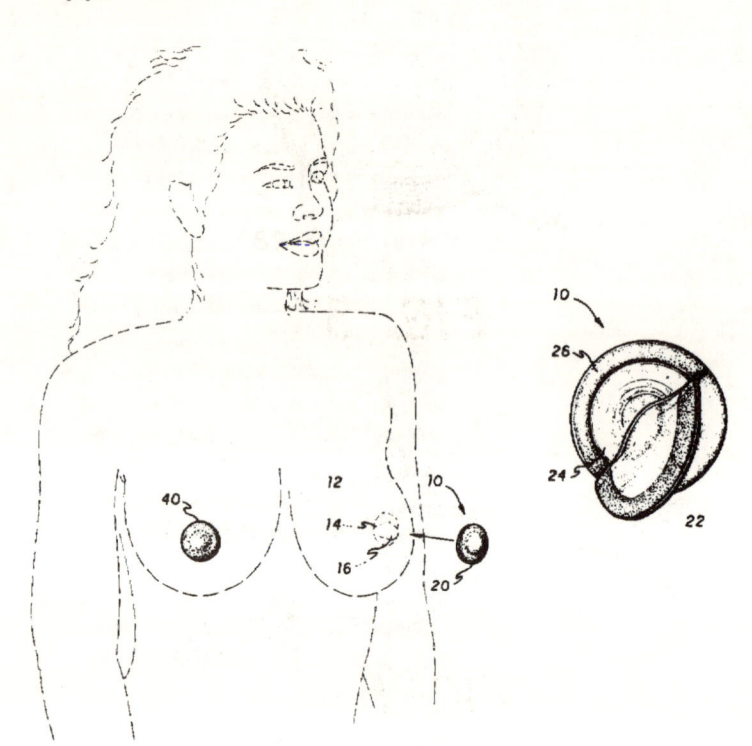

## Abstract

A nipple pad for protecting and concealing the nipple and areola of a woman's breast includes a pliable cover, a padded liner, adhesive strips, and a release liner. The padded liner is affixed to a central portion of the cover. The adhesive strips are attached to the periphery of the cover, concentrically surrounding the padded liner. The release liner is attached to the adhesive strip for covering and protecting both the adhesive strip and the padded liner. The central portion of the cover and the padded liner have a concave shape for receiving the nipple, resulting in enhanced contouring and softening thereof. The padded liner has an increasing thickness from the periphery to the central portion of the cover, resulting in maximum contouring and softening of the nipple.

FIG. 2

FIG. 3

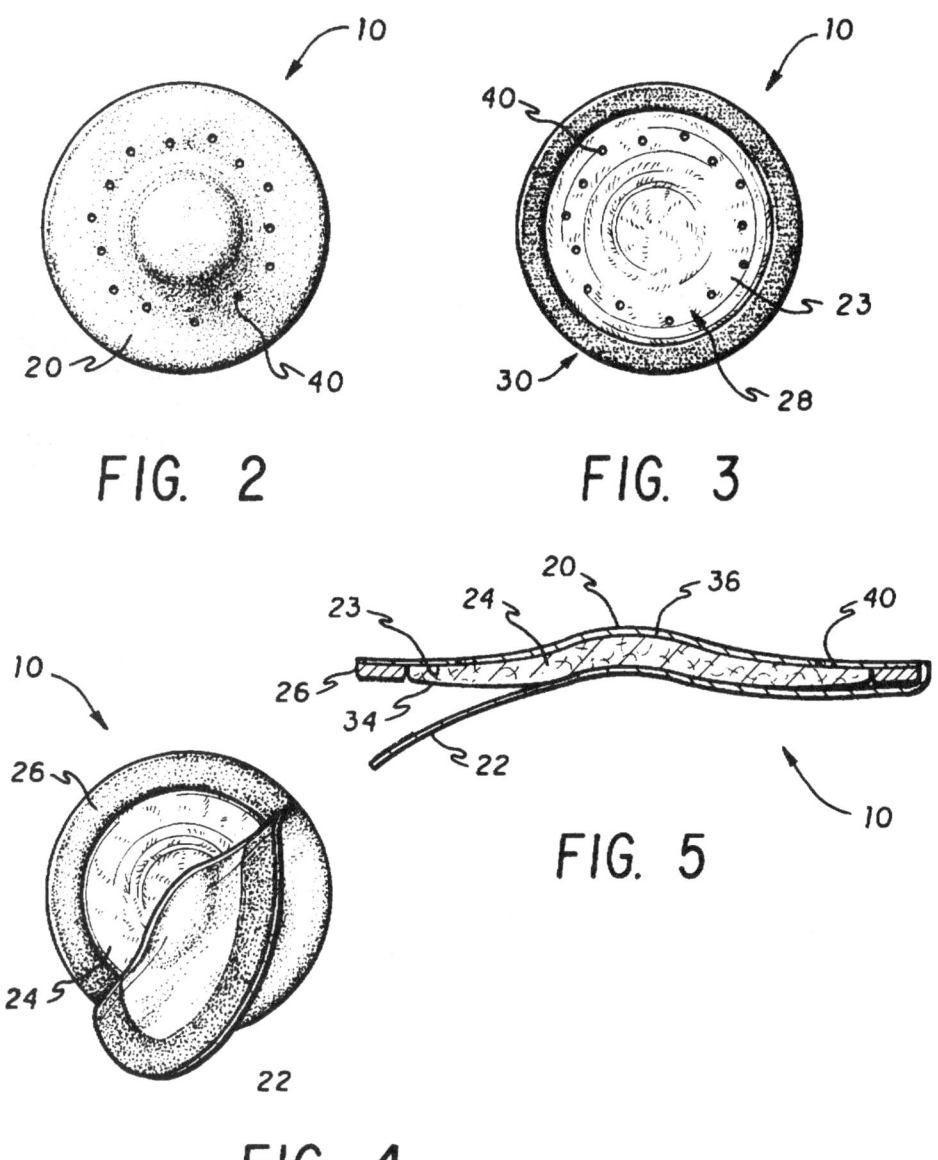

FIG. 4

FIG. 5

Patent No. 4,949,731
Aug 21, 1990
Glen R. Harding

# Oral Prophylactics

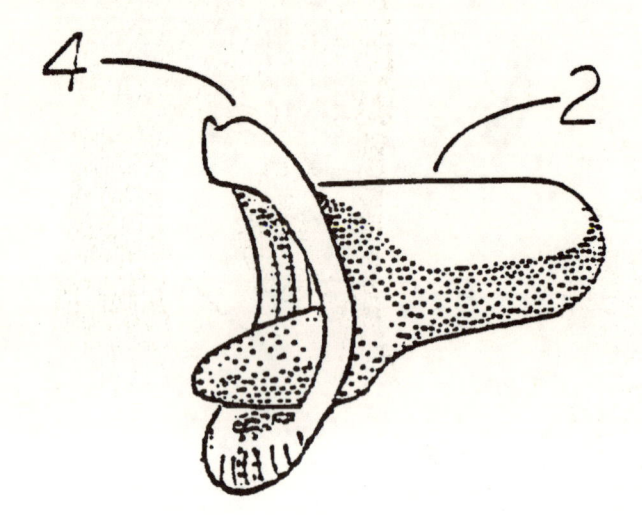

### Abstract

An elastic and flexible oral prophylactic that conforms to the mouth. The hygienic appliance may incorporate texture and flavor, and includes impermeable and permeable embodiments.

FIG 1

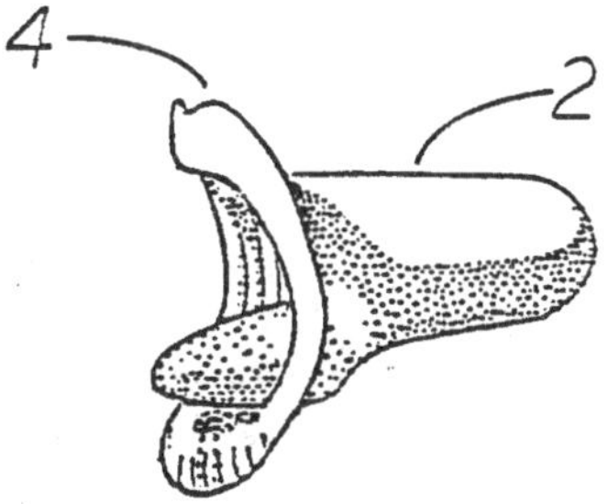

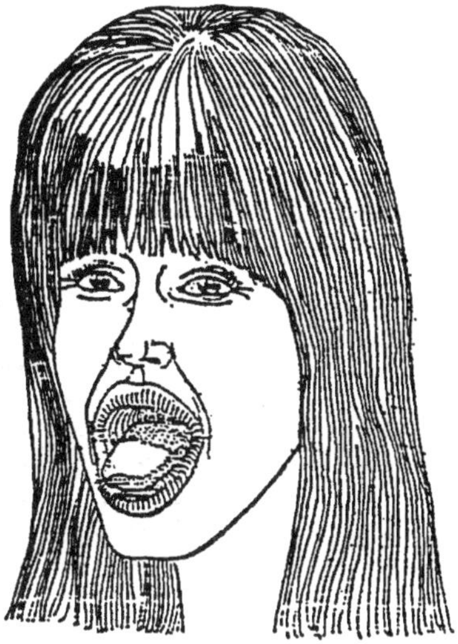

FIG 2

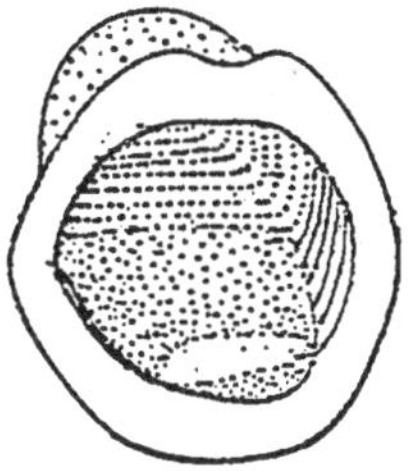

FIG 3

FIG 4

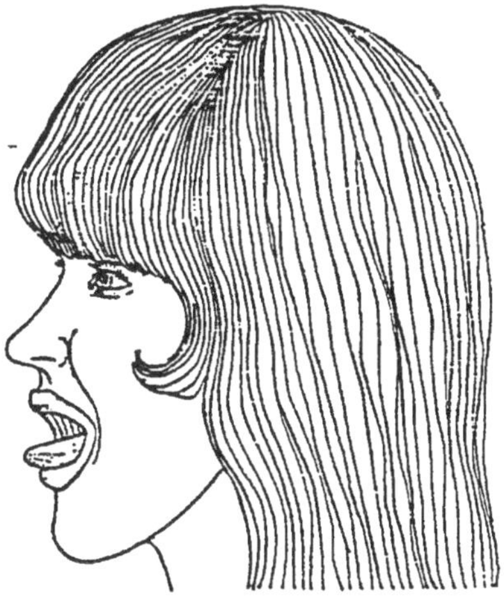

FIG 5

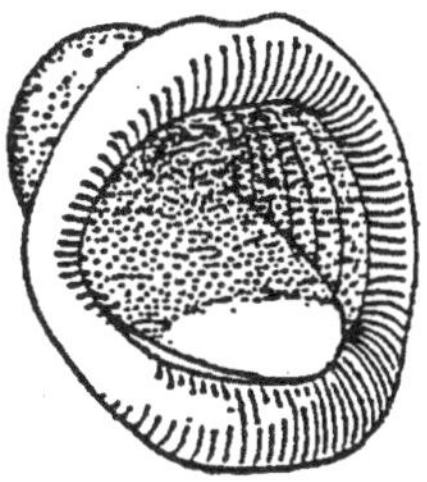

FIG 6

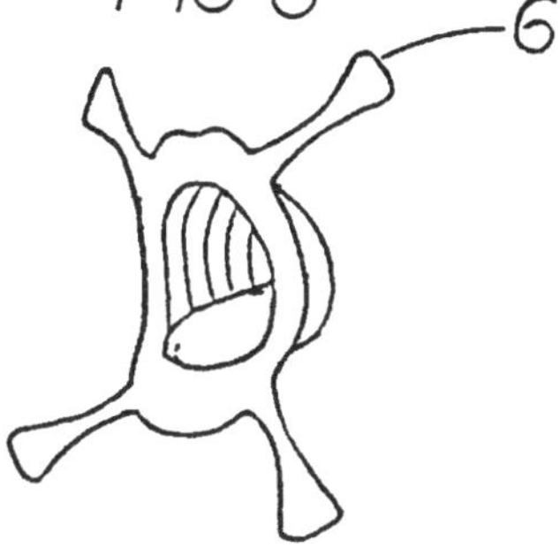

# Panty Condom

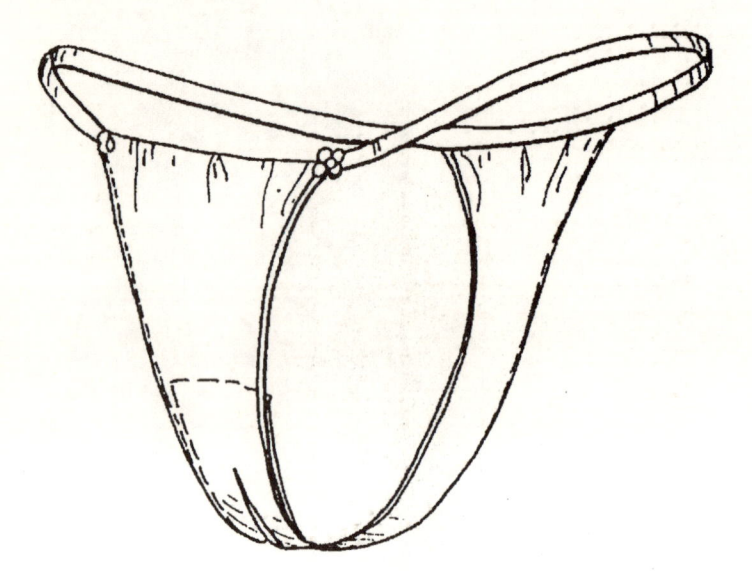

Patent No. 5,596,997
Jan 28, 1997
Max M. Abadi

## Abstract

A female panty condom having an opening generally at the genital area of the wearer and located approximately over the vagina of the wearer. A pouch including a front side having a slit and a back side having a slit is affixed to the panty such that the opening in the panty, the slit in the front side of the pouch and the slit in the back side of the pouch are aligned. A sheath is positioned within the pouch behind the slit in the front side of the pouch such that the penis of a male partner may enter the opening of the sheath through the opening in the panty. The sheath will extend to cover the penis as it moves through the slit in the back side of the pouch and into the vagina of the wearer.

FIG.1　　　　　　　　　FIG.6　　　　　　　　　FIG.7

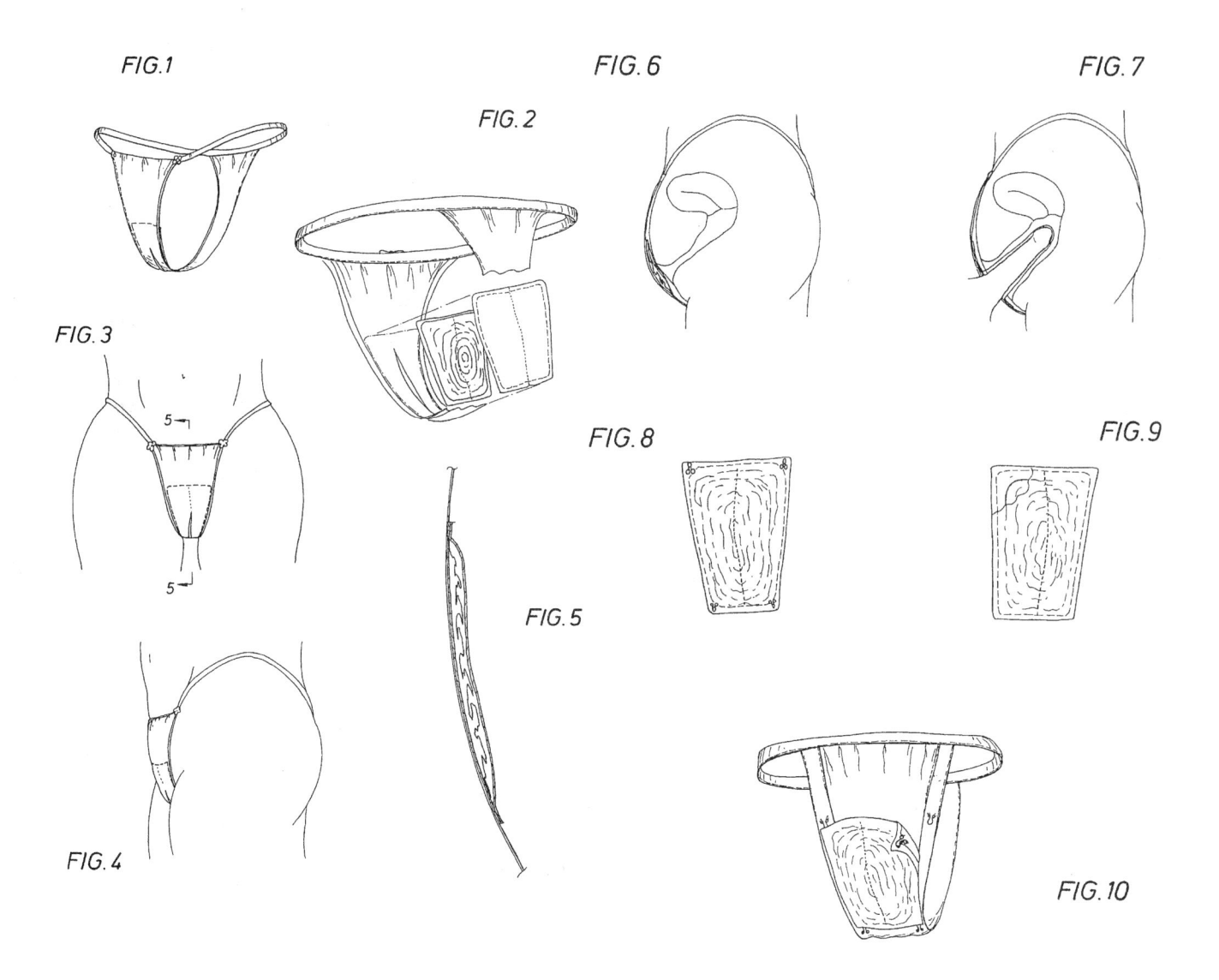

FIG.2

FIG.3

FIG.5　　　　FIG.8　　　　　　FIG.9

FIG.4　　　　　　　　　　　　　　FIG.10

97

Patent No. 4,653,484
Mar 31, 1987
Lamar J. Cannon

# Penile Erection Aid

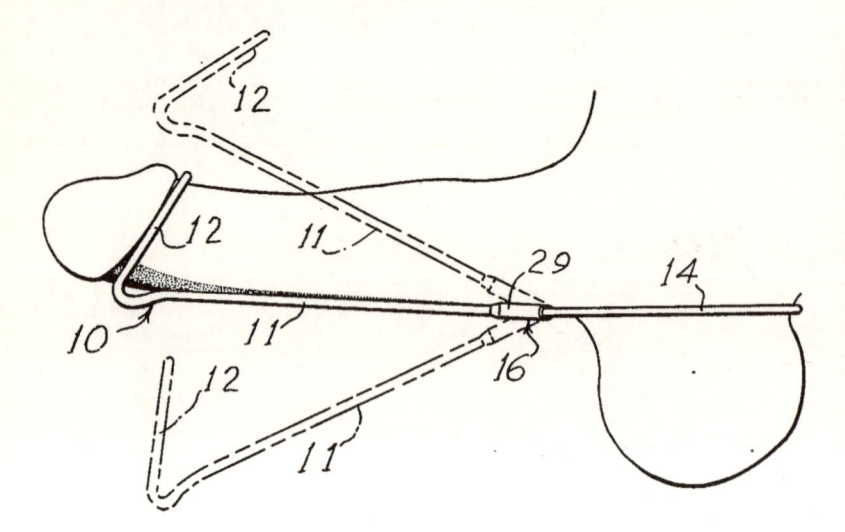

## Abstract

A penile erection aid for assisting a flaccid or partially flaccid penis in penetration. The device includes a splint held to the underside of the penis, with an anchoring ring fixed to the splint and passing around the penis at the base of the extremity. The inner end of the splint is hinged to an anchoring ring that passes around the scrotum, the anchoring ring being held in place by straps. The pair of straps connected to the front of the anchoring ring can be crossed to exert pressure at the base of the penis to assist in maintaining a partial natural erection.

Fig. 1

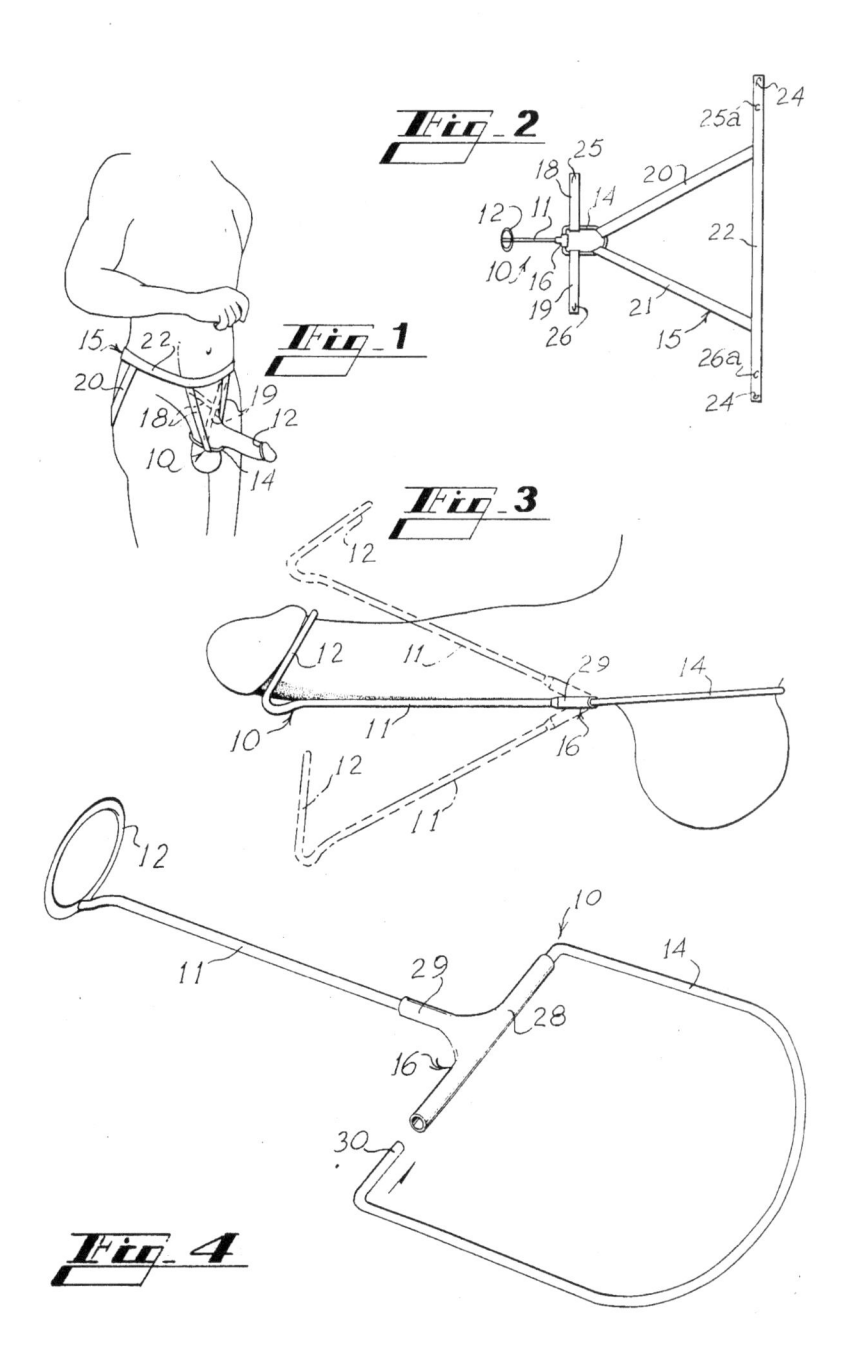

Fig. 2

Fig. 3

Fig. 4

Patent No. 4,022,196
May 10, 1977
Robert E. Clinton

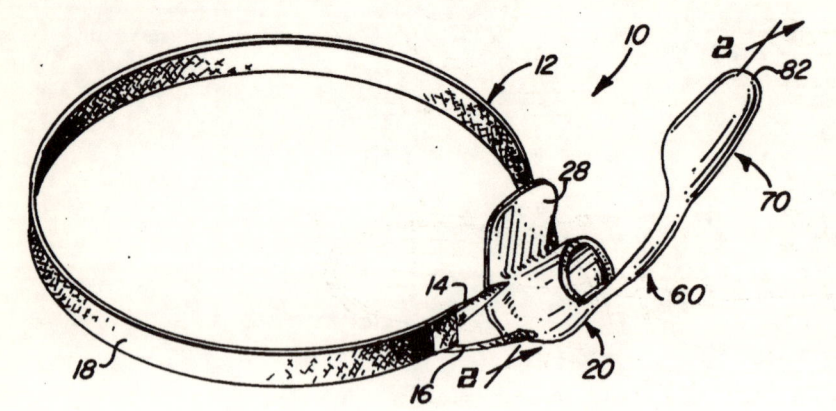

# Penile Prosthetic Apparatus

### Abstract
Penile prosthetic apparatus which includes a relatively rigid base to support the apparatus against the male body and into which fits a male penis for enhancing male and female sexual relations.

FIG-1

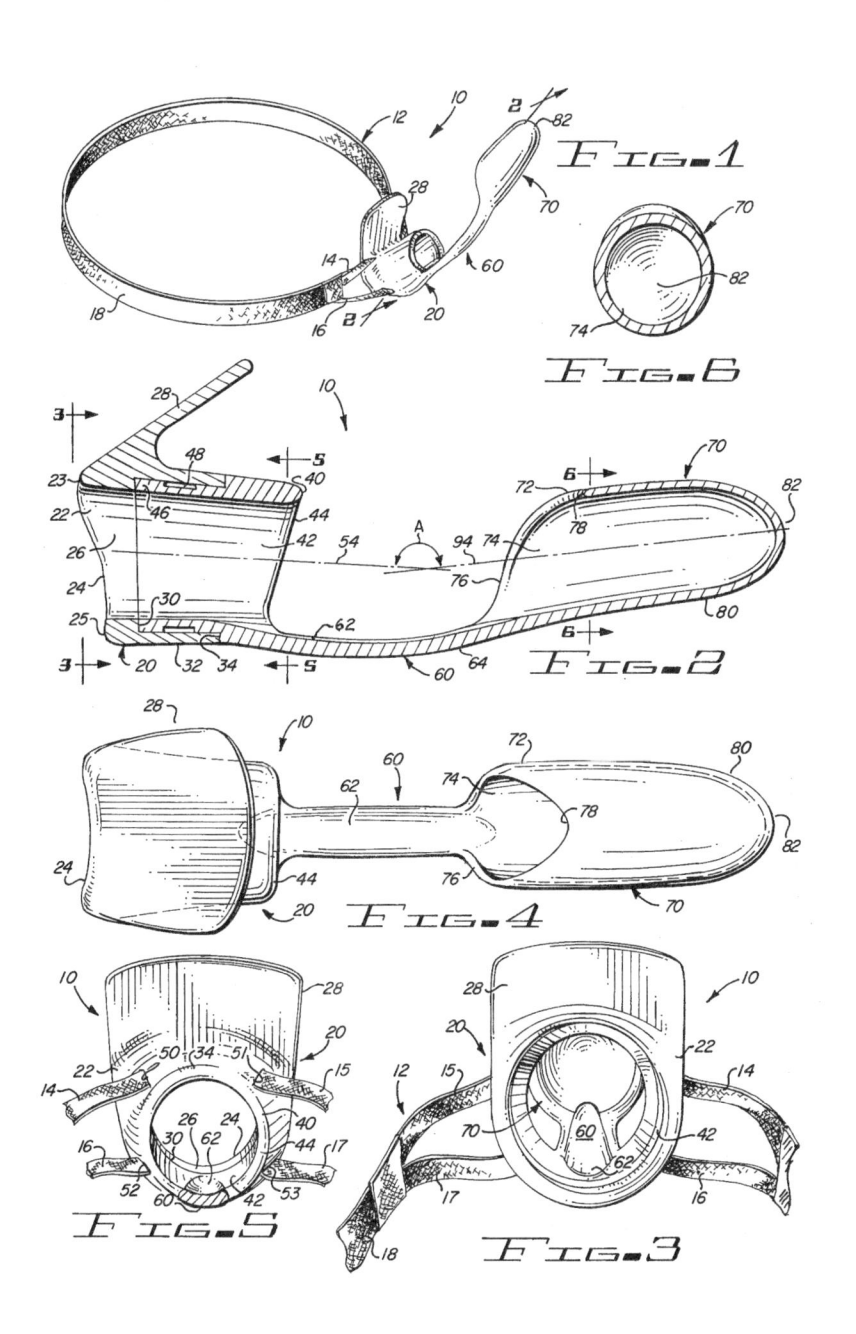

FIG-6

FIG-2

FIG-4

FIG-5

FIG-3

101

Patent No. 1,346,463
July 13, 1920
John J. Renois

# Penis Surgical Splint

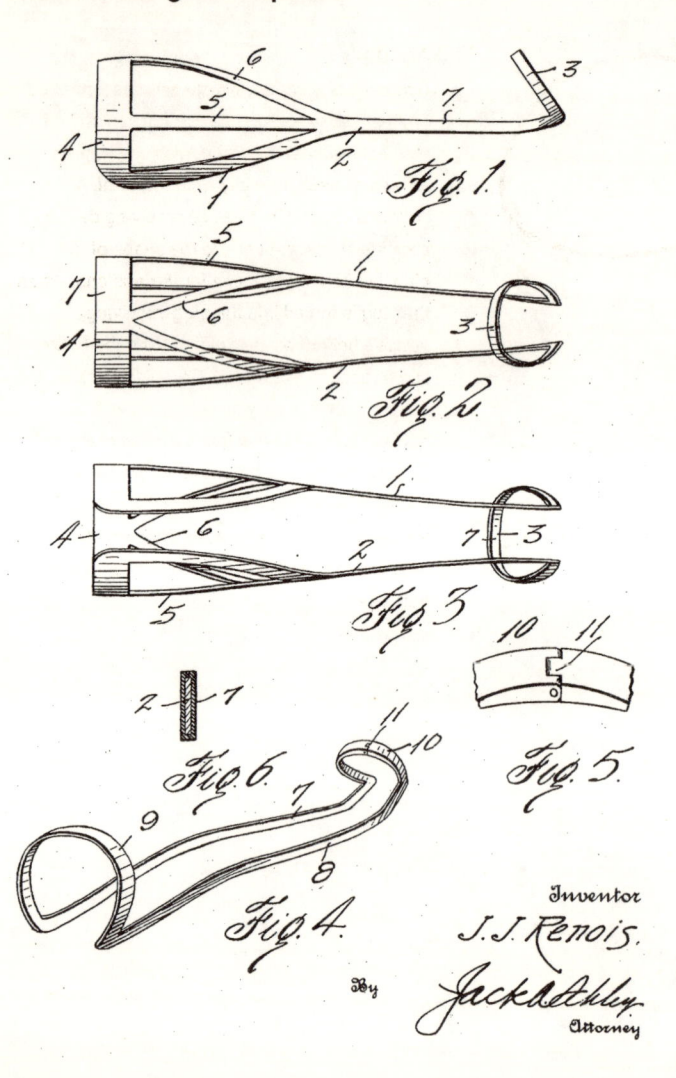

## Abstract

This invention relates to improvements in self sustaining splints. The invention has to do with a mechanical substitute for the erectile tissue of the corpora cavernosa of the genital organ so that fecundation may result even in the absence of an erection. An elongated resilient member is provided with supporting loops at each end and capable of transverse adjustment to fit the organ to which it is applied.

Patent No. 5,127,396
July 7, 1992
Ron McAllister

## Plug and Phallic Device and System

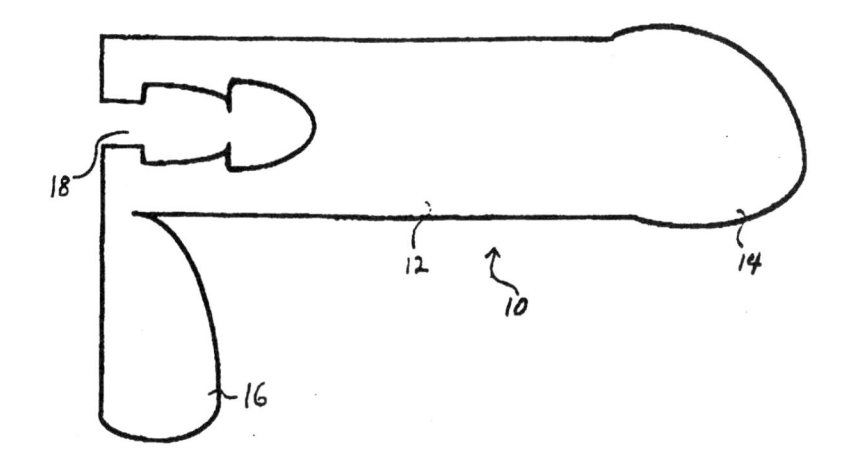

### Abstract

Disclosed is a system which includes a phallus or other plug-receiving device formed of resilient material in combination with a plug formed of a substantially rigid material. A hollow is shaped in the plug-receiving devices' back which corresponds to the shape of the plug, but has slightly smaller dimensions. When the plug is forced into the plug-receiving device's hollow, air is expelled from the hollow and a vacuum-like fit is achieved. Preferably, the plug and phallus may be combined with a harness formed of inelastic clothlike material forming the body of the harness, the body having a length sufficient to reach around from the wearer's lower abdomen, between the wearer's legs and up onto or over the wearer's buttocks.

Patent No. 3,991,751
Nov 16, 1976
Jessie O'Rourke

# Portable Vibrator

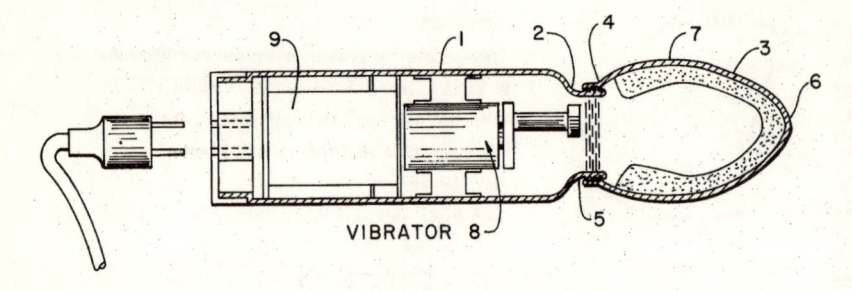

### Abstract
A tubular housing is dimensioned to be held in a hand and has an open neck end. The housing has a predetermined diameter throughout its length and a diameter smaller than the predetermined diameter at the neck end thereof and is rounded down at its neck end from the predetermined diameter to the smaller diameter. An electric vibrating device in the housing vibrates the head.

Patent No. D246,119
Oct 18, 1977
Tadao Okamoto

## Prophylactic Device (Condom)

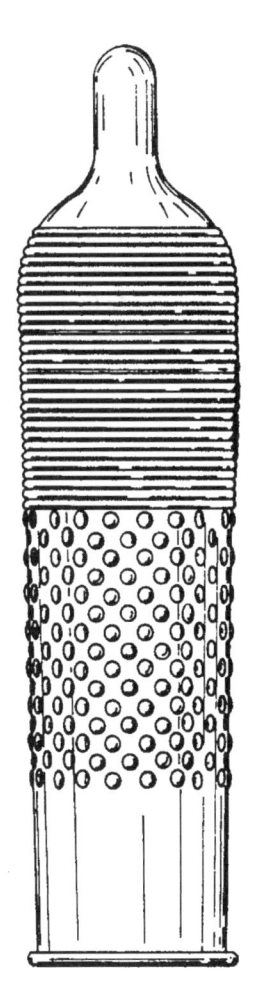

### Abstract

The ornamental design for a prophylactic device, as shown. This is an elevational view of a prophylactic device showing my new design. Also a top plan view thereof and a bottom plan view thereof.

FIG. 2

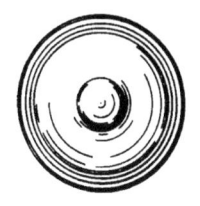

FIG. 3

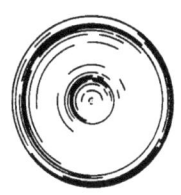

Patent No. 4,807,611
Feb 28, 1989
Kenneth A. Johnson

# Prophylactic Device (Underwear)

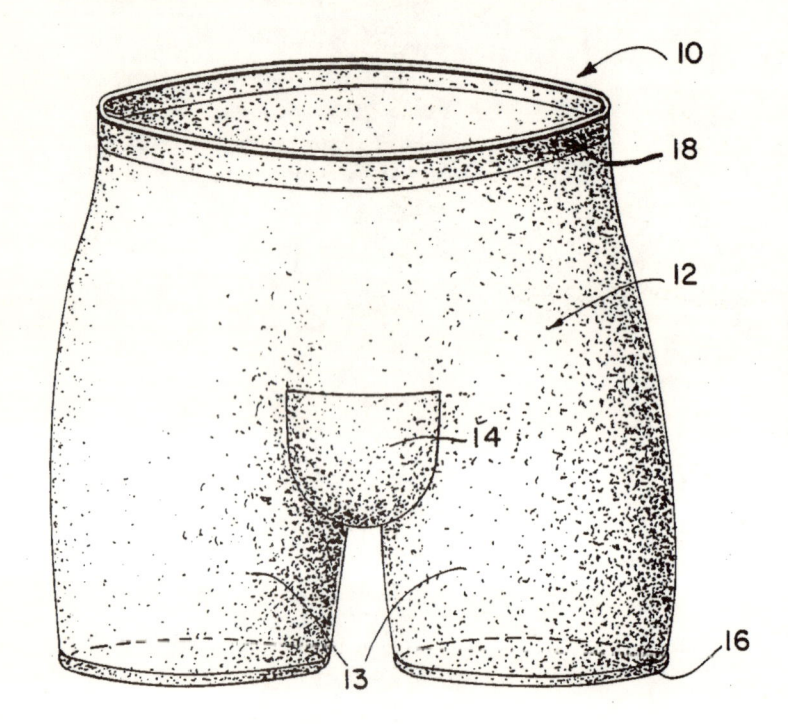

## Abstract

A prophylactic device designed to isolate completely those portions of the body most susceptible to the introduction of infected bodily fluids of another into the bloodstream. The device includes a body portion fitting the wearer like a garment, extending from the vicinity of the navel downward to extend onto the thighs. A trap portion, either integral with or fixed to the body portion, covers the perineum of the wearer. The latter portion is formed of a highly expandable material and fitted loosely. The trap portion can respond to pressure from within or without to extend outwardly or inwardly to maintain an impermeable barrier between a penetrating member and the interior of a target office.

*FIG. 2.*

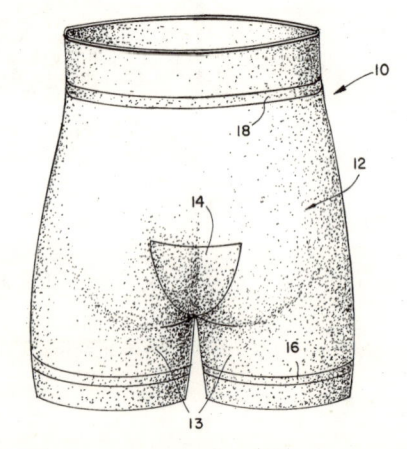

FIG. 3.

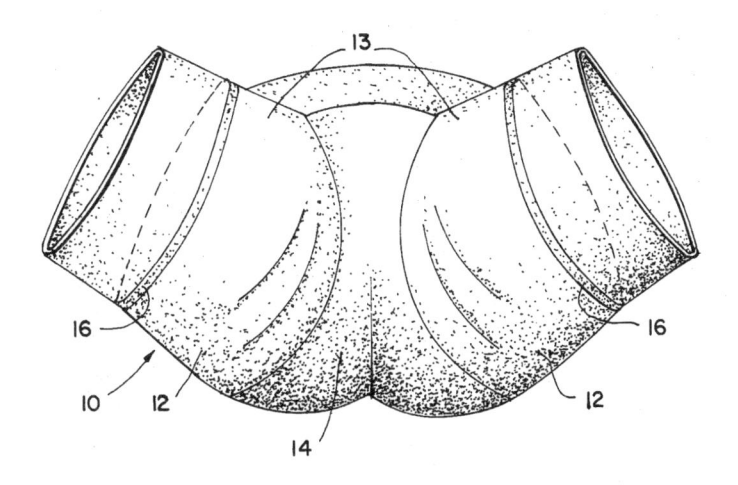

FIG. 4.

# Prostate Gland Massaging Implement

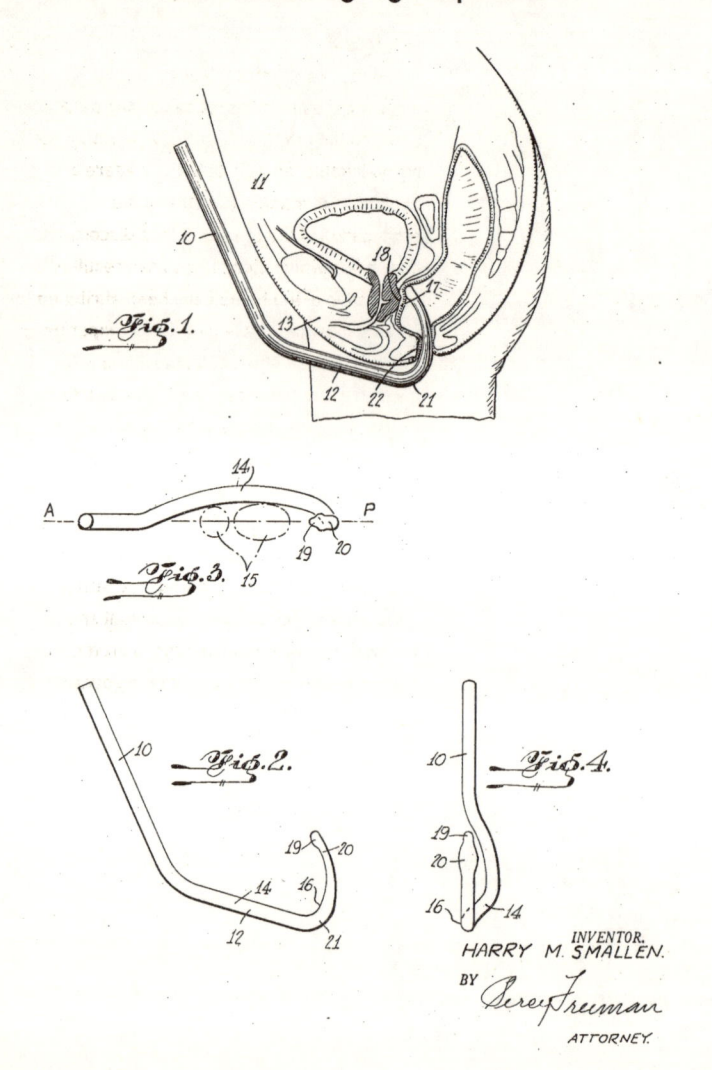

Patent No. 2,478,786
Aug 9, 1949
Harry M. Smallen

## Abstract

This invention relates to an instrument for the treatment of the prostate gland and has especial reference to an implement for massaging said gland. It is known that material benefit may be obtained in prostate gland cases by the gentle massage of the gland. Such cases usually require the attendance and attention of a physician mainly because there has been no suitable instrument or implement by which a patient, upon instruction and under the direction of his physician, may accomplish his own treatment or massage of the gland. Then, too, because of lack of adequate implement for the purpose, the time of a physician was required for the treatment of such cases when his time could be better employed in handling more urgent cases which do not lend themselves to self-treatment by the patient.

Patent No. 2,899,957
Aug 18, 1959
John J. Briggs

# Prosthetic Appliance

FIG. 1

FIG. 2

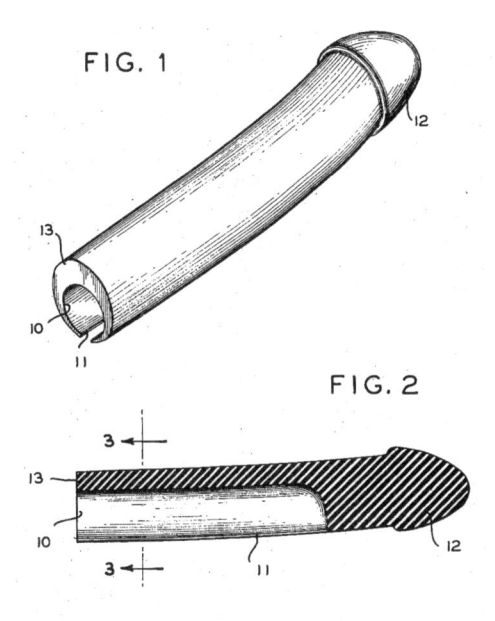

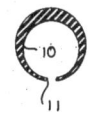

FIG. 3

INVENTOR
J. J. BRIGGS

BY *A. Yates Dowell*
ATTORNEY

## Abstract

This invention relates to human relations including the promotion of peace and harmony between the sexes and particularly within the marital status, as well as to the welfare and happiness of mankind, including the propagation of the species. While discord and dissension which sometimes have resulted in destruction of the home have been attributed to various reasons, I have found from experience that difficulties between husband and wife frequently are because of tensions resulting from unhappiness caused by frayed nerves brought on by failure of one or the other to maintain a calmness notwithstanding a lack of satisfaction. An object of the invention is to bridge the chasm between the sexes, particularly husbands and wives suffering from a malevolent lack of mental, spiritual and physical complementation, and to promote the marital relations and the mutual enjoyment of the beautiful of life.

Patent No. 5,582,187
Dec 10, 1996
Cynthia L Hussey

## Protective Mask

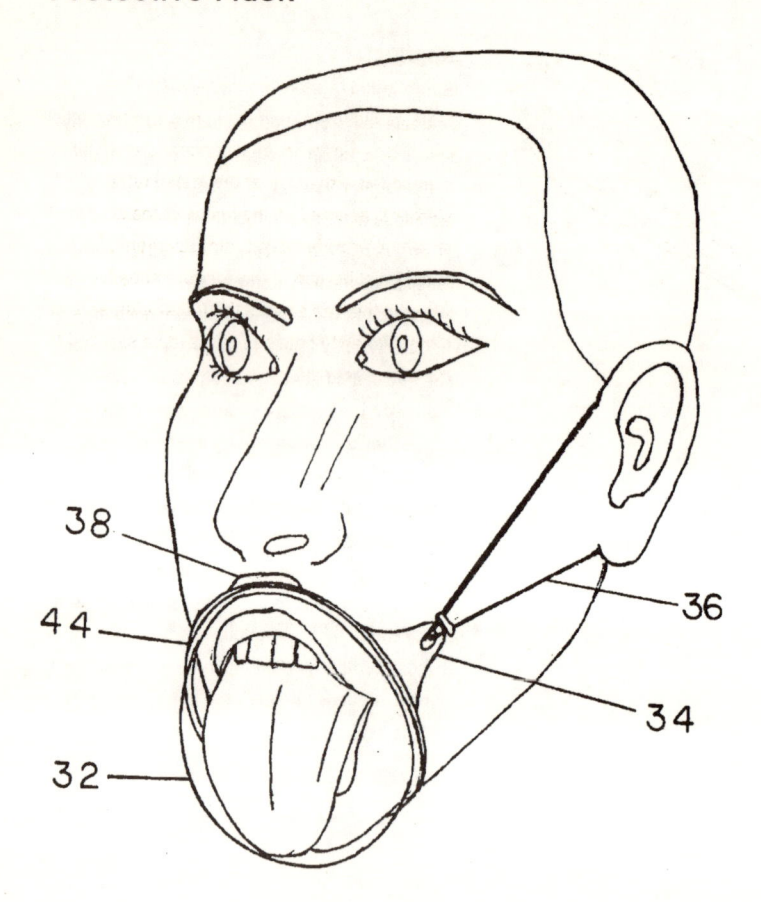

### Abstract
A thin, flexible shield for the mouth to protect against transmission of STDs (Sexually Transmitted Diseases) during cunnilingus and oral-anal sex. A shield is held over the mouth either alone or in a holder assembly by mounting devices which retain the mask against the face of the user. The holder assembly may consist of one or two rings interlocked with each other or with the shield to grip the shield.

Patent No. 5,121,755
June 16, 1992
Joseph Hegedusch

# Reinforced Tethered Condom Construction

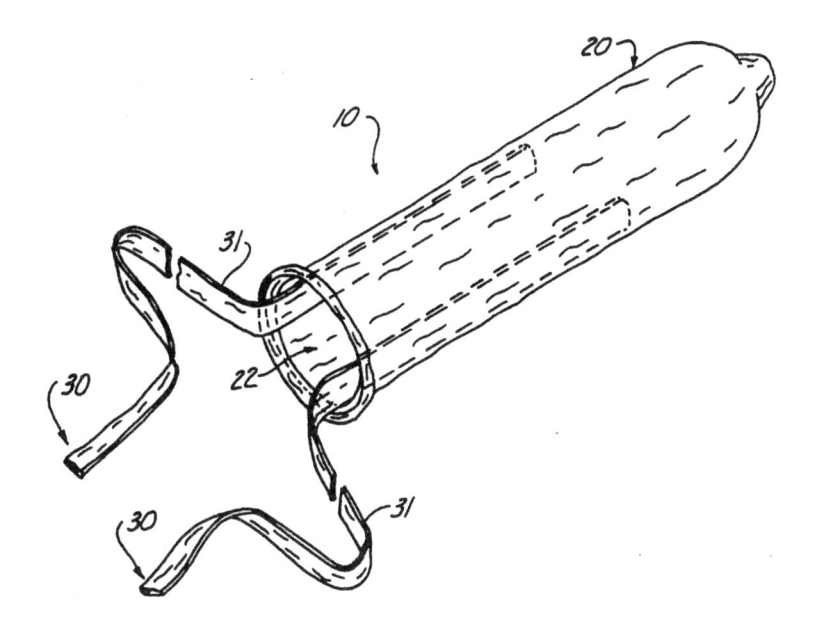

## Abstract

A reinforced tethered condom construction for male genitalia wherein the condom construction comprises a conventional condom sheath which is provided with a pair of elongated tether elements secured on the inside of the condom sheath to provide lateral reinforcement along a substantial portion of the condom sheath and wherein the free ends of the tether elements are dimensioned to both encircle and be secured to the user's genitalia.

# Rolling Ring Condom

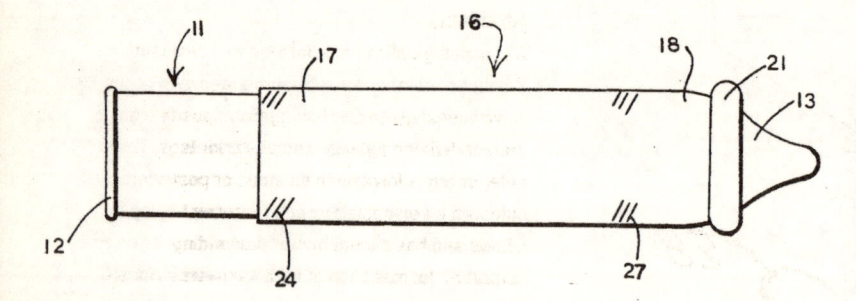

Patent No. 5,425,379
June 20, 1995
Robert L. Broad Jr.

## Abstract

A contraceptive device having a condom that has a configuration of an elongated tube having an open end and a closed end. A sheath surrounds at least a portion of the tubular condom. The sheath has an attachment end and a distal end. The attachment end of the sheath is attached to the condom at a first point. The distal end of sheath is located at a second point spaced from the first point. An elastic ring is secured to the distal end of the sheath. The sheath is unattached to the condom between the points such that the elastic ring is free to move back and forth between the points.

Patent No. 3,996,930
Dec 14, 1976
Mark W. Sekulich

## Self-Contained Gynecologic Stimulator

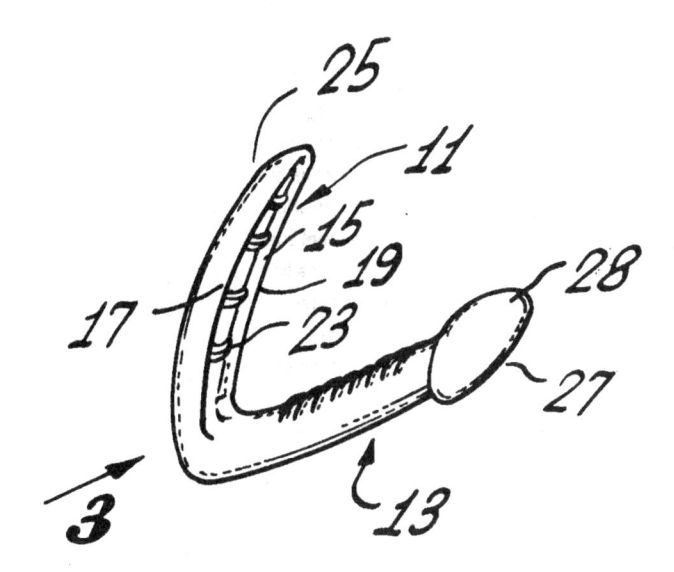

### Abstract

A gynecologic stimulator formed by a resilient V-shaped member for receipt in a wearer's vulvovaginal gland and having the opposite legs thereof defining anterior and posterior legs. The anterior leg is formed on its inner, or posterior, side with an elongated trough for receipt of the clitoris and has a longitudinally extending central rib formed therein with transverse rings spaced therealong.

# Sensory Transmitting Membrane Device

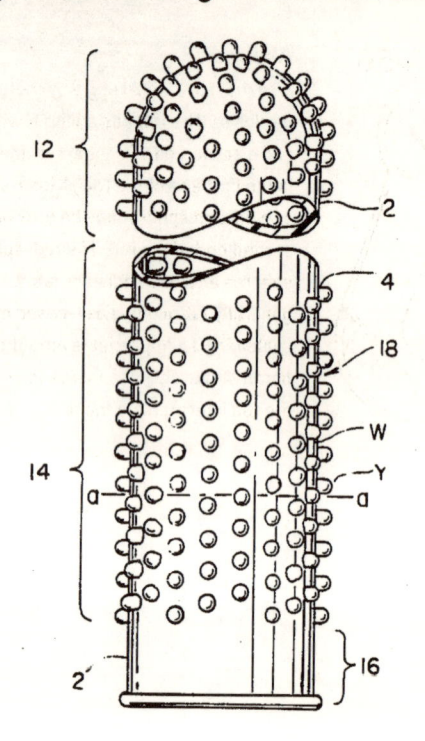

Patent No. 4,852,586
Aug 1, 1989
Bernard M. Haines

## Abstract

A device for the transmission and enhancement of tactile sensations transmitted across a barrier membrane, particularly condoms, finger cots and gloves used to prevent transmission of disease organisms between contacting body tissues. The device has a plurality of antipodal pairs of projections extending through the barrier membrane whereby the barrier membrane acts as a fulcrum for the transmission of movement by one projection of an antipodal pair to the other member of the projection pair.

Patent No. 6,132,366
Oct 17, 2000
Steven D. Ritchie; Harlie David Reynard

# Sex Aid

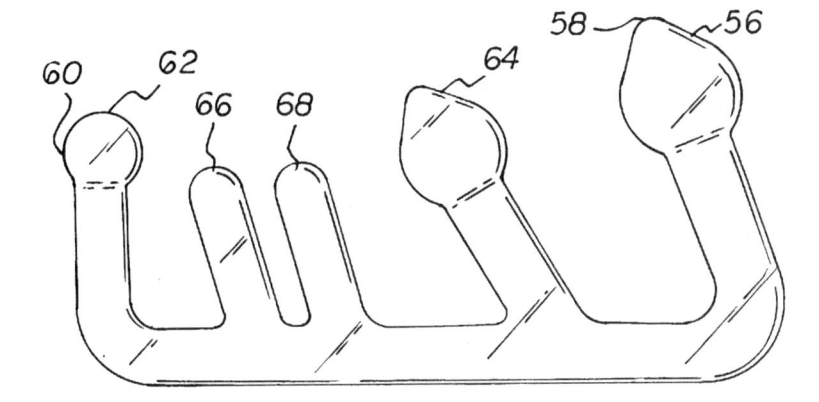

### Abstract

A sexual aid comprising a cylindrical rod is disclosed. The rod has a length with a first end and a second end. A sphere is integrally formed in the first end of the rod. A loop-shaped handle or a second sphere may be provided on the second end of the rod. The rod, sphere or spheres and/or handle are fabricated of a generally lubricous glass-based material containing an appreciable amount of an oxide of boron. A plurality of spheres may be provided on the rod intermediate the first and second ends.

# Sex Aid Device for Males

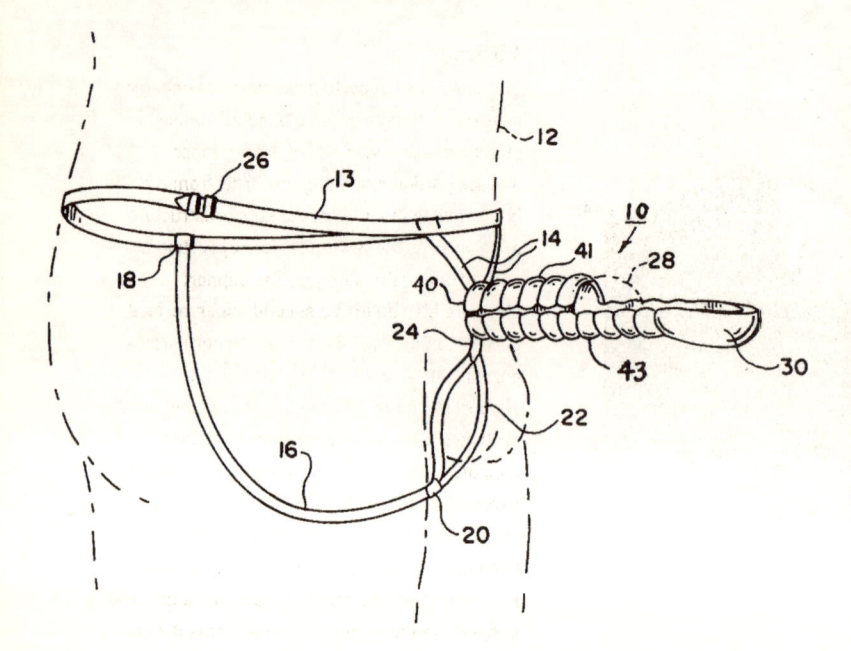

Patent No. 4,429,689
Feb 7, 1984
Procopio U. Yanong

## Abstract

A sex aid device for males is disclosed comprising a tubular member that includes upper and lower longitudinally extending relatively inelastic but flexible supports and connecting elastic flexible sides, said tubular member being adapted to extend from the base of a penis to the glans penis, and the bottom support extending forward and forming a relatively inelastic spoonlike member for receiving the bottom of the glans penis to be exposed to tactile stimulation, said spoonlike member having a forward-extending smooth tip of soft compressible elastic material formed thereon.

Patent No. 3,855,652
Dec 24, 1974
Dana C. Nicholson

## Sex Couch

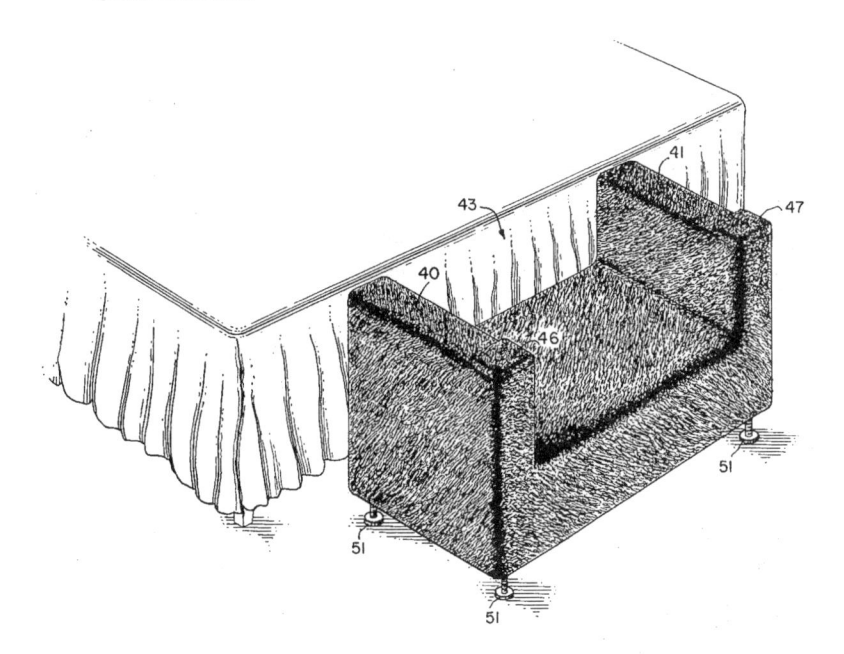

### Abstract

In a couch for supporting two persons engaging in sexual intercourse, an elongated support structure is provided having a first upper surface portion extending upwardly from a point intermediate the ends of the support structure at an angle to the horizontal for supporting the back of one of the persons. The support structure also defines a second upper surface portion connecting with the first upper surface portion with a recess being formed in the support structure and dividing the second upper surface portion into two spaced arms for supporting the legs of the above mentioned one person. The recess is located and dimensioned in a manner to accommodate the other person in a kneeling position between the spaced arms. In a second embodiment, for use with a bed, the support structure comprises two arms divided by a recess. The height of the arms is selected to correspond to the height of a bed.

Patent No. 5,725,473
Mar 10, 1998
Larry Thornell Taylor

# Sexual Aid

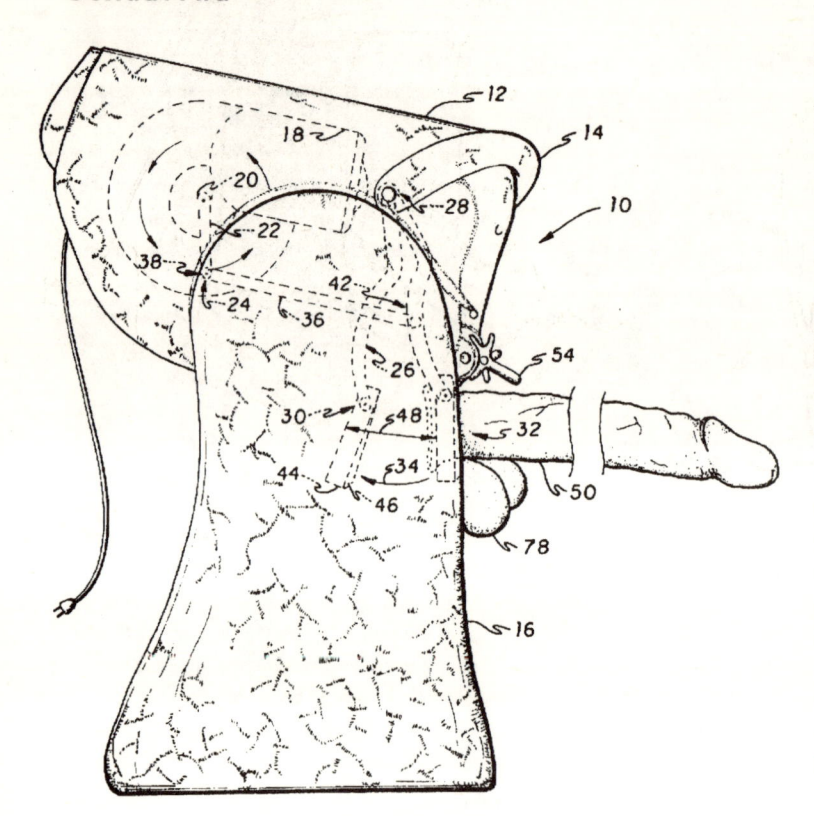

### Abstract

A sexual aid including a housing, mounted on detachable legs and containing a motor that urges a dildo, including vibration means, to describe an arcuate path generally coincident with an orifice, such as a vagina. A first stimulator, also containing vibration means, is superposed above the dildo and is urged through an arcuate path concentric with and radially spaced inwardly from that of the dildo, cyclically contacting a clitoris. The sexual aid may include means for introducing a vacuum between the first stimulator and the clitoris. A second stimulator, also containing vibration means, is subjacent to the dildo and is urged through an arcuate path concentric with and radially spaced outwardly from that of the dildo, cyclically contacting an anus. The sexual aid includes remotely locatable stimulators that may be placed in contact with a user's nipples and areolae. The sexual aid also provides a vacuum phenomenon between the remotely locatable stimulators and the nipples.

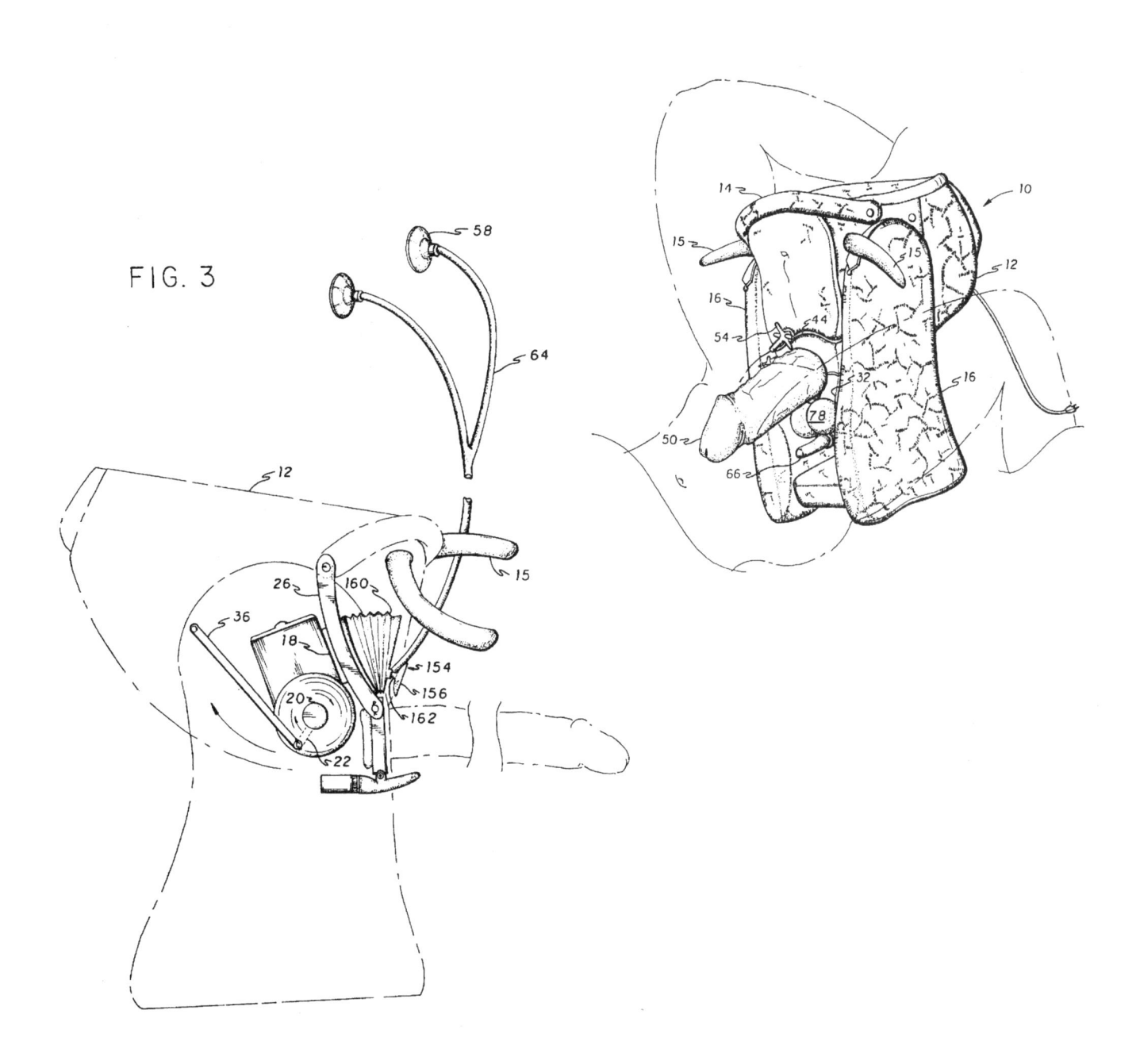

FIG. 3

119

Patent No. 5,997,469
Dec 7, 1999
Michael E. Northcutt

## Sexual Aid Device

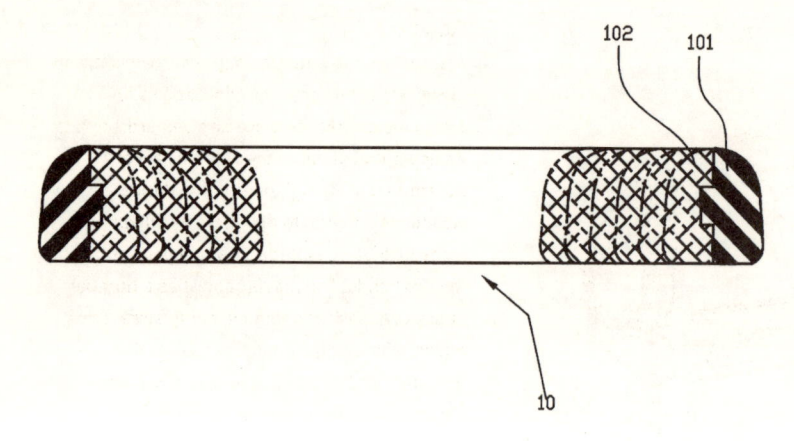

### Abstract

A sexual aid device that encircles the base of the penis. The device may be constructed as a single ring, or as a set of rings that can be used together in various conformations. The device includes a size adjustment means that allows the user to vary the size of the central through hole so that a user of the device is always ensured of a proper fit. The device may also include an extension means to directly stimulate the female's clitoral region. Alternatively, the device may be formed with an oval shape as opposed to a round shape to achieve the objective of direct stimulation of the clitoris.

Patent No. 5,103,810
Apr 14, 1992
Tao-Ping Chang

## Sexual Aid (Strap-On)

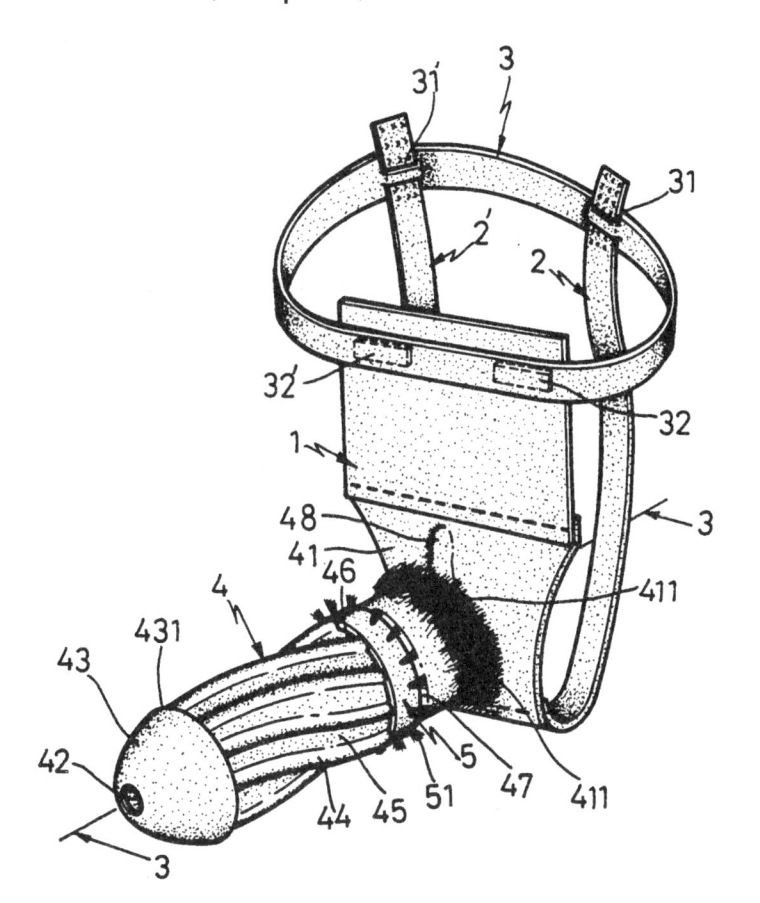

### Abstract

A sexual aid has a tubular body with a connection piece, two bands sewn or adhered to a lower end of the connection piece and a guard sewn to an upper end of the connection piece. For adjustment of the tightness of the device, a waistband adhered to the guard by adhesive tapes defines slots through which pass ends of the two bands. The tubular body has a number of peaks and valleys running along spiral lines which, with a ring element, stimulate the woman in order to make her reach orgasmic phase more quickly. The tubular body is a hollow structure with a hole at the front end to allow sperm to flow therethrough.

Patent No. 5,693,002
Dec 2, 1997
Martin Tucker; Fai Pang Lin;
Serafin Antonio Hernandez

# Sexual Appliance Having a Suction Device Which Provides Stimulation

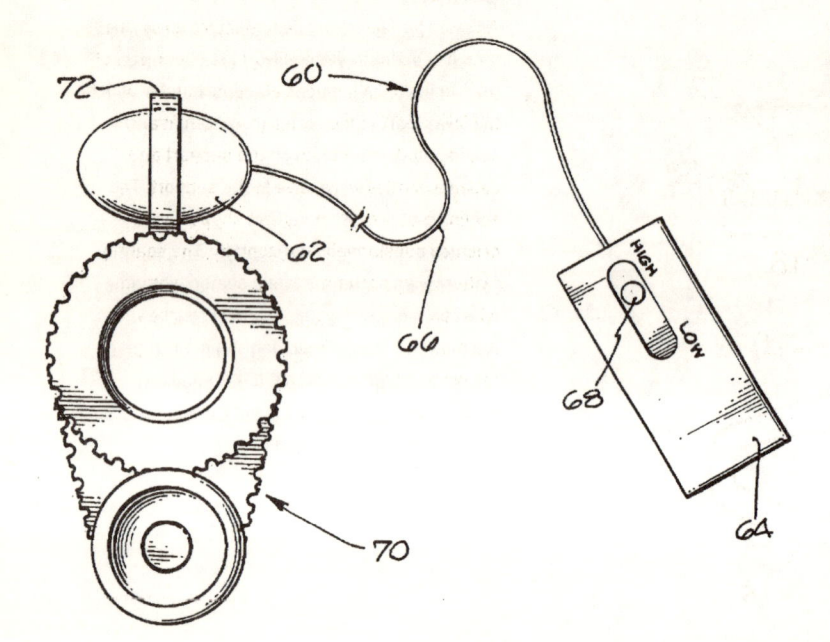

## Abstract

A sexual appliance that includes a main body portion having an aperture adapted to receive the wearer's penis and a suction device associated with the main body portion and adapted to apply a suction force to a predetermined portion of the anatomy of the wearer's intercourse partner.

Patent No. 5,294,176
Mar 15, 1994
Ruven Asinovsky

# Sexual Device for Handicapped Men

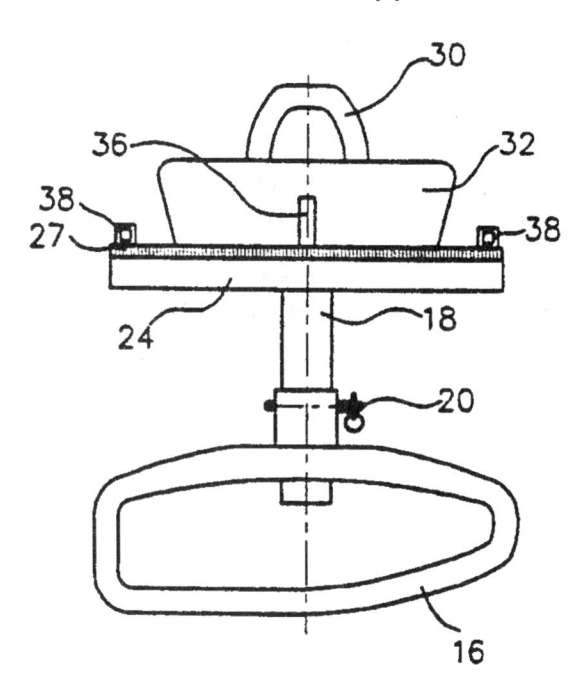

### Abstract

A device for facilitating sexual intercourse of a man having limited mobility of the lower part of the trunk, which includes a support under which the lower part of the man's trunk can fit and a seating platform resting on the support and capable of rotation relative to the support. The seating platform is annular in shape and is oriented substantially horizontally. The seating platform can accommodate a seated woman who can thereby have sexual intercourse with the man without the man bearing the weight of the woman and without his having to exert motions of the lower part of his trunk.

Patent No. 4,641,638
Feb 10, 1987
Robert D. Perry

# Sexual Erection Prosthesis and Method of Use

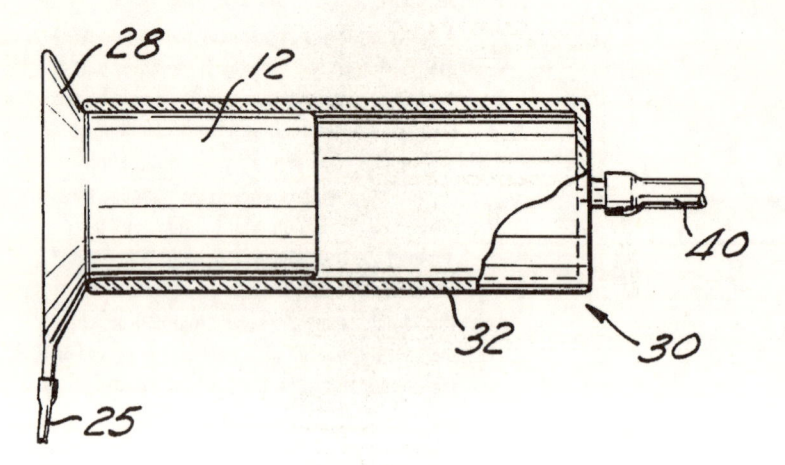

## Abstract

A sexual erection prosthesis and method of use is disclosed adapted to artificially activate and maintain the penal [*sic*] erection state in human males. The system includes a flexible relatively supple prosthetic device which is sized to encircle the male penis and incorporates an expansible diaphragm adapted to provide localized constrictive engagement against the penis. The system additionally includes an artificial vascularization assist device which is utilized in combination with the tubular member to obtain hydraulic blood pressure within the penis as well as an insertion device to aid in the placement of the device upon a penis. The system permits the rapid release of the constriction at a desired time to prevent self-injury to the user.

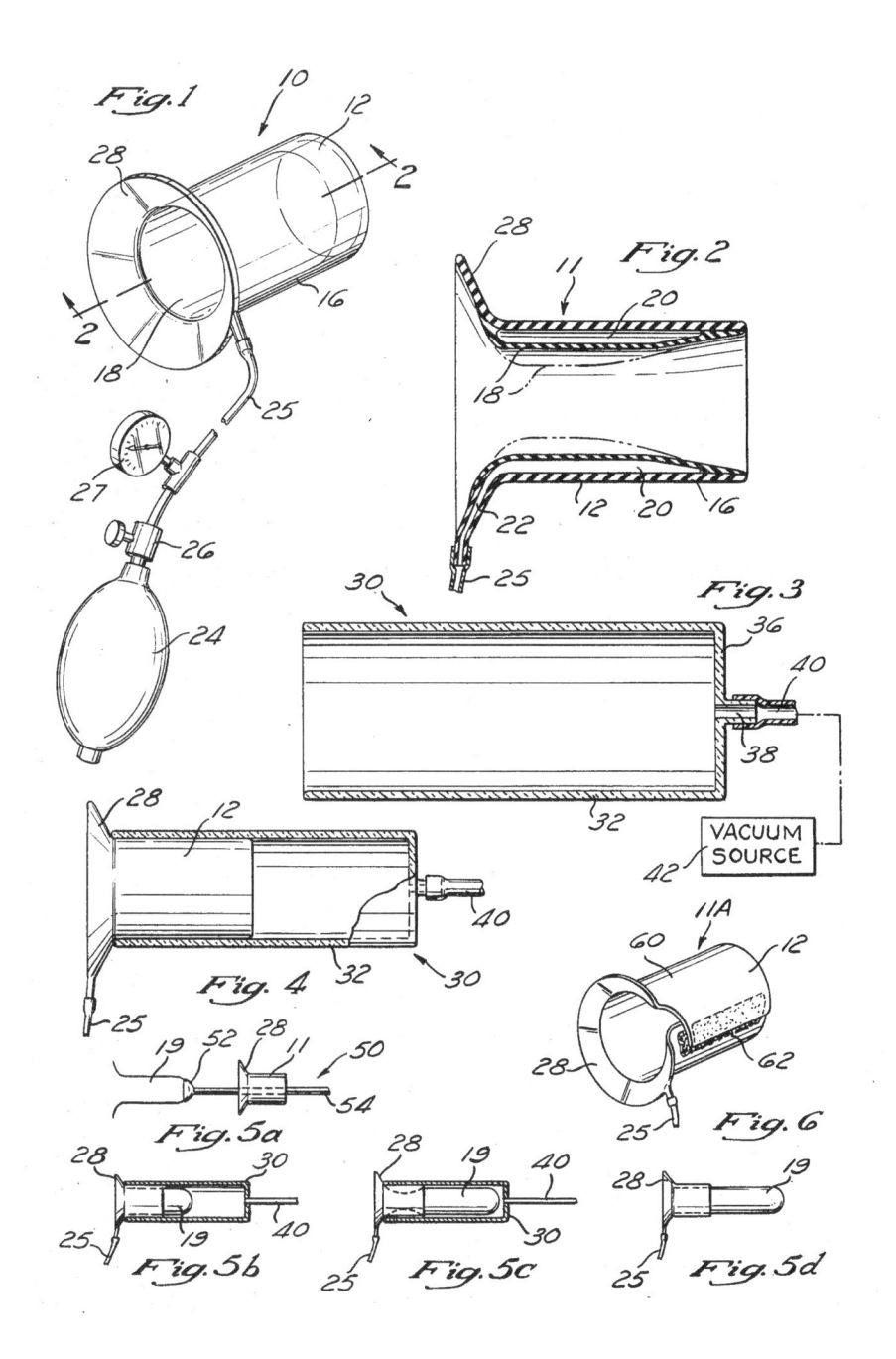

Fig. 1
Fig. 2
Fig. 3
Fig. 4
Fig. 5a
Fig. 5b
Fig. 5c
Fig. 5d
Fig. 6

Patent No. 6,142,929
Nov 7, 2000
George Glenn Padgett

# Sexual Stimulation Apparatus

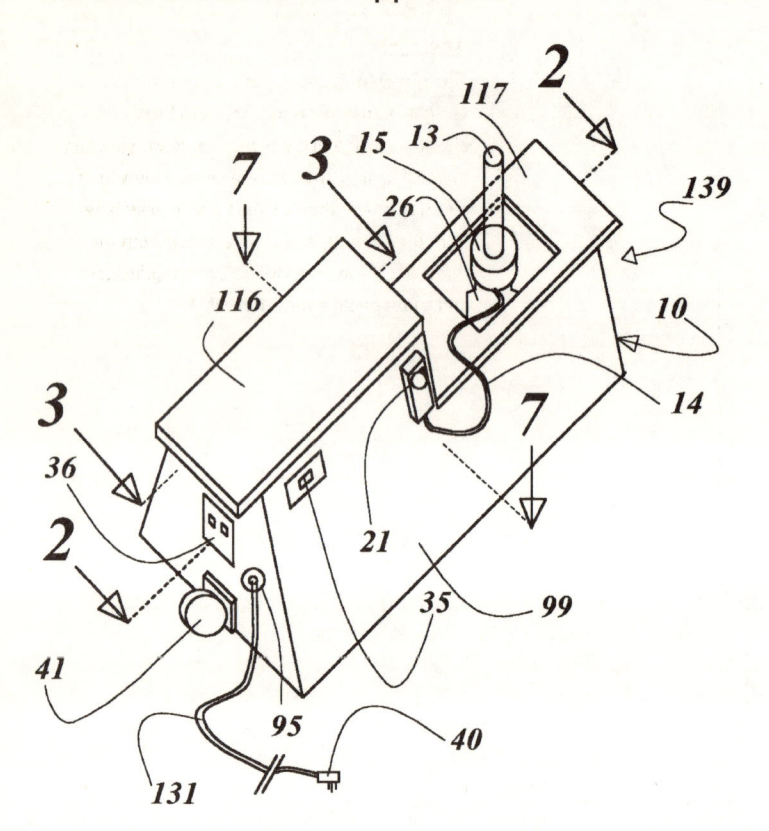

### Abstract

A sexual stimulation apparatus for the sexual gratification of a woman or man, by stimulating vaginal or anal intercourse, which generally includes a long hollow box or tube; with a seat for two persons on top; inside the container mechanical levels and cranks powered by an electric gear reduction motor; an on/off switch; a power indicator light; a ground fault interrupt circuit; a rheostat; and a dildo mounted on the end of a lever which is positioned underneath the seat so the dildo extends through a hole in the seat and thrusts in a generally vertical motion. The commercially obtained, vibrating or non vibrating dildo, can be of various shapes, girths, lengths and textures, and may or may not be remotely controlled.

# Sexual Stimulator

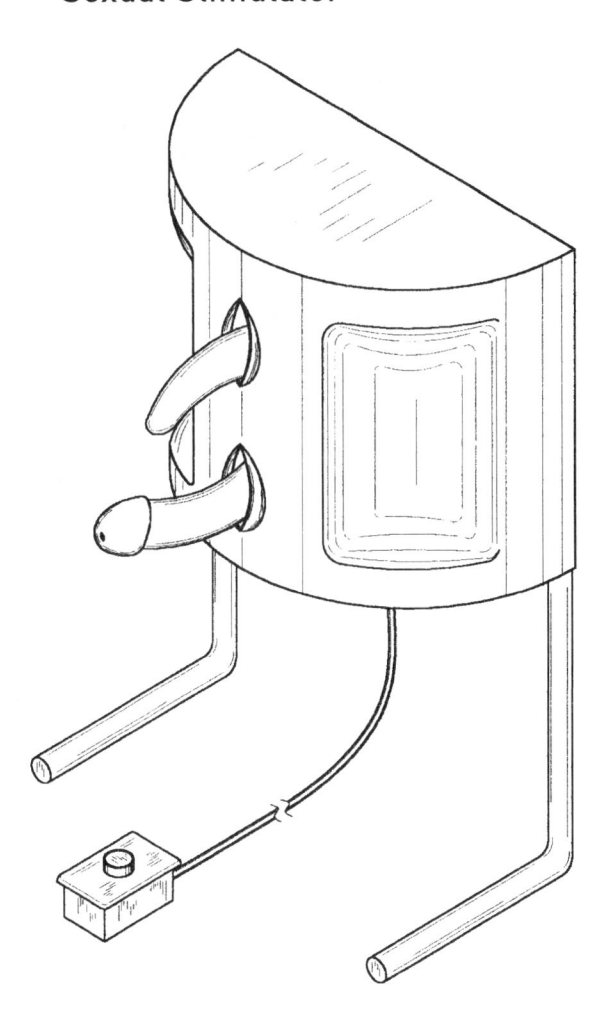

Patent No. US D466,218 S
Nov 26, 2002
Shawn M. Dalton

## Abstract

The ornamental design for a sexual stimulator, as shown and described. This is a front elevational view of a sexual stimulator showing my new design, the rear elevational view being a mirror image thereof. Also a side view taken from the left side, a side view taken from the right side, a top plan view, a bottom plan view, and a perspective view thereof.

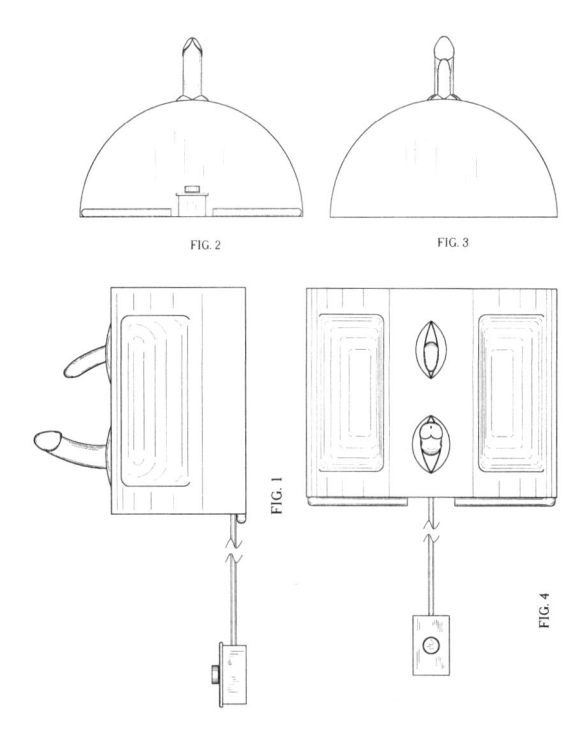

FIG. 2

FIG. 3

FIG. 1

FIG. 4

Patent No. US 6,490,732 B1
Dec 10, 2002
Conrad Spoke

# Spreader Means Garment

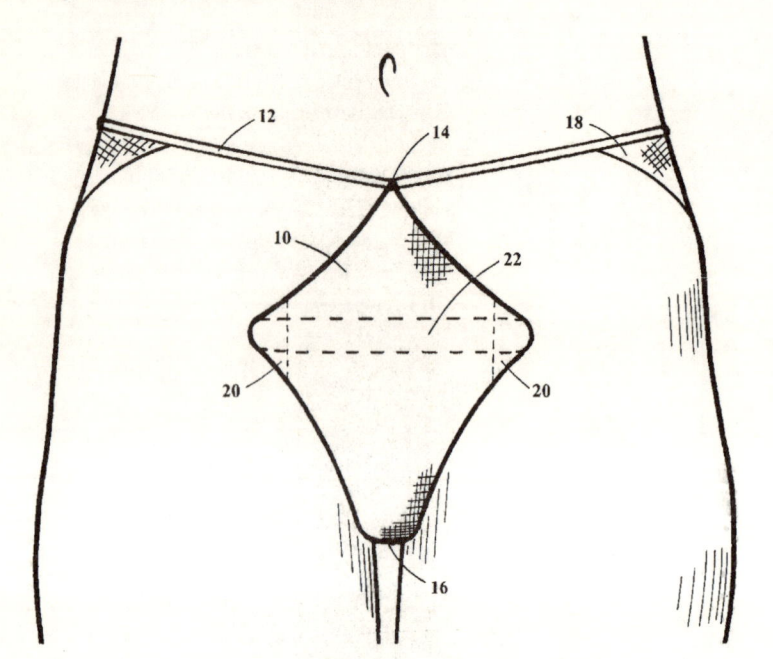

## Abstract

A bikini-style swimsuit having a diamond-shaped cloth pubic panel, and a spreader which communicates with restraining pockets. The spreader extends the left and right extremities of the panel, tensing the cloth in the horizontal axis. A waistband and a crotch panel of typical bikini construction tense panel in opposing directions in the vertical axis. An unexpected synergy of forces compels the entire periphery of the diamond-shaped panel to be pulled into contact with the body of the wearer in an attractive and modest fashion.

Fig. 1

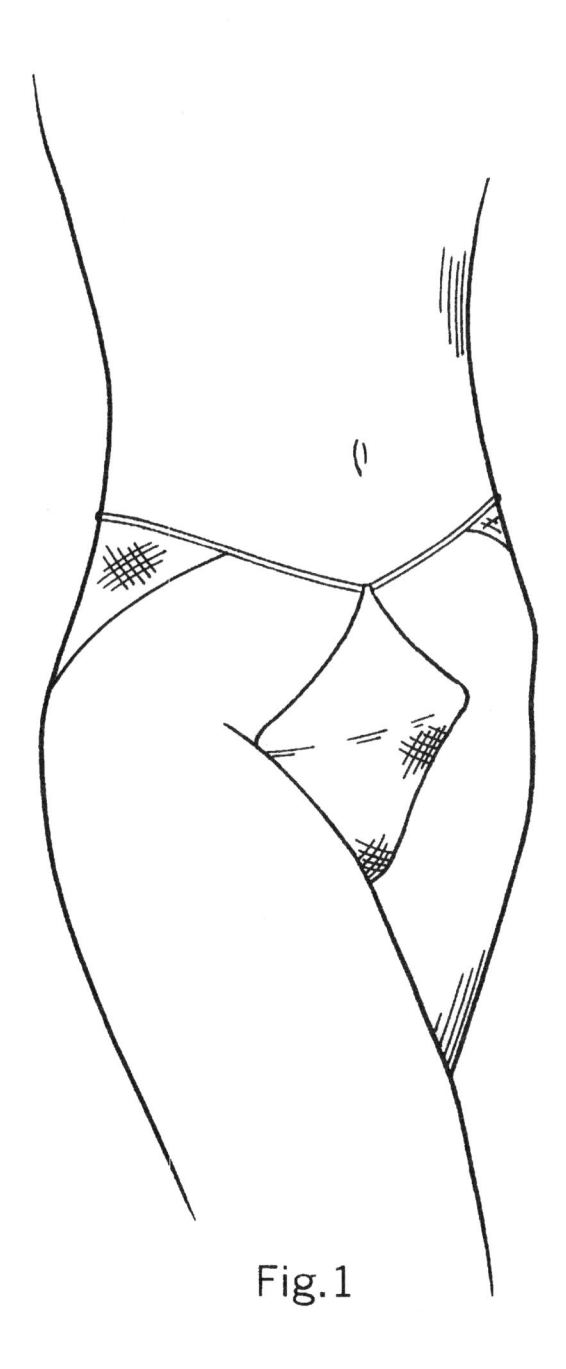

# Stimulator

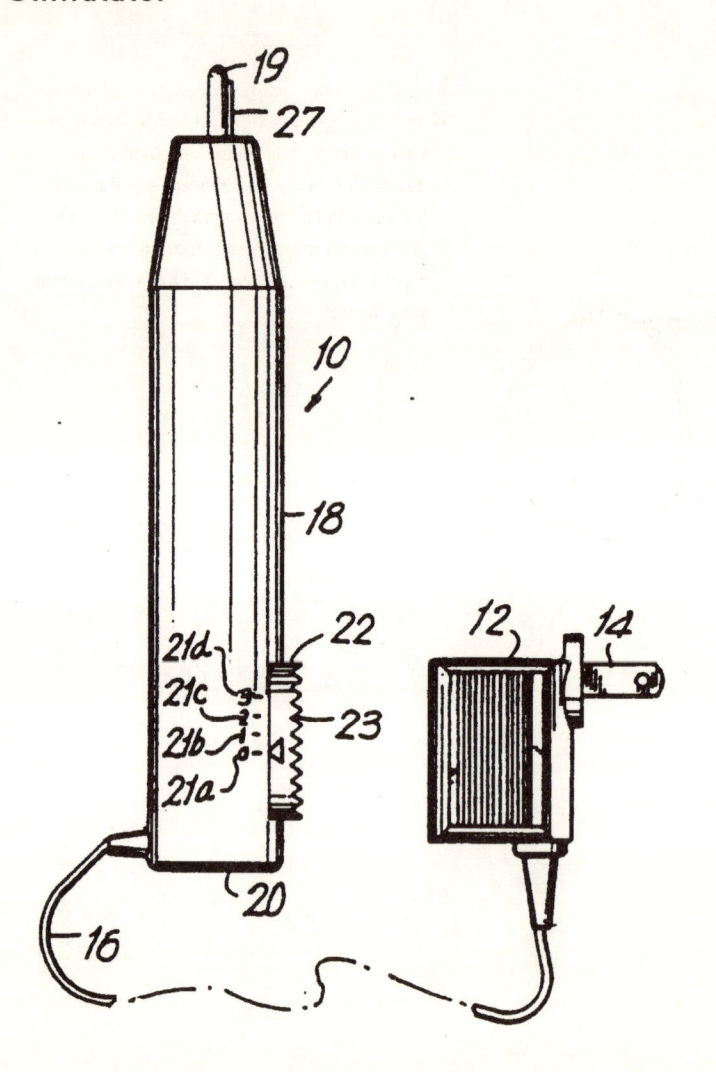

Patent No. 5,067,480
Nov 26, 1991
Philippe-Guy E. Woog; Michael A. Moret

## Abstract

A stimulator for use in marital orgasmic therapy is provided. The stimulator uses a step-down transformer and a water-proof case. The stimulator oscillates at 2000–8000 (preferably 3000–3600) cycles per minute throughout an angle of operation chosen from the range of 10 to 80 (preferably 20 to 60) degrees. An integrated set includes several different detachable attachments and a handle with mechanical oscillating means.

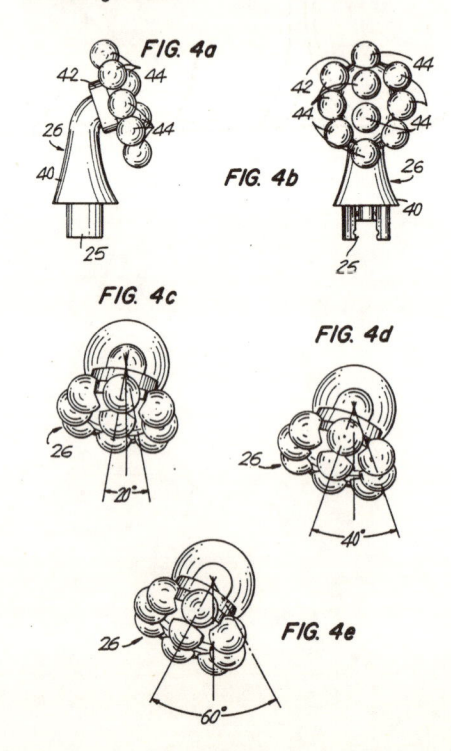

Patent No. D395,081
June 9, 1998
Frederick John Bowden

# Strap On Condom

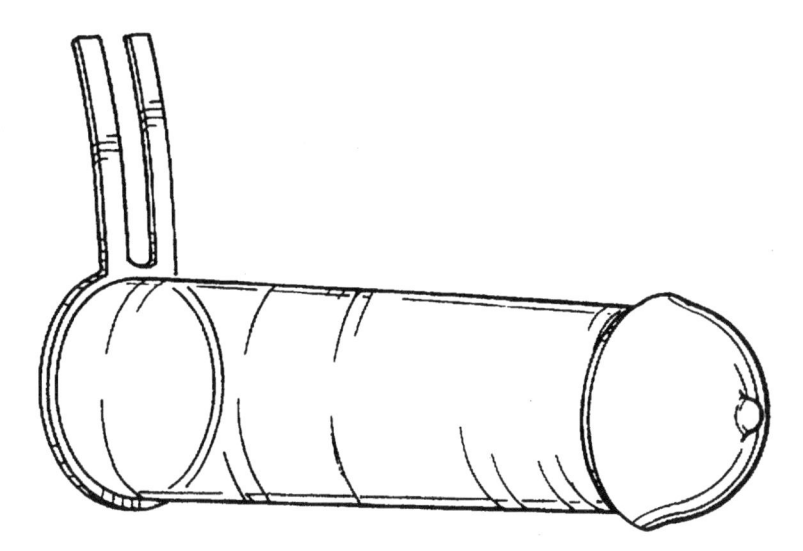

## Abstract

The ornamental design for a strap on condom, as shown and described. This is a perspective view of a strap on condom, showing my new design. Also a top view thereof; a bottom view thereof; a left side elevational view, the right side being a mirror image thereof; a front elevational view thereof; and a rear elevational view thereof.

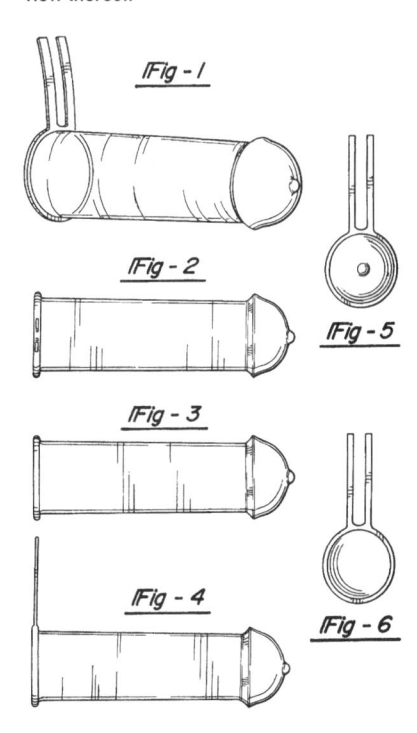

*Fig - 1*

*Fig - 2*

*Fig - 3*

*Fig - 4*

*Fig - 5*

*Fig - 6*

Patent No. 5,531,230
July 2, 1996
Ray W. Bell

# Strap Secured Condom

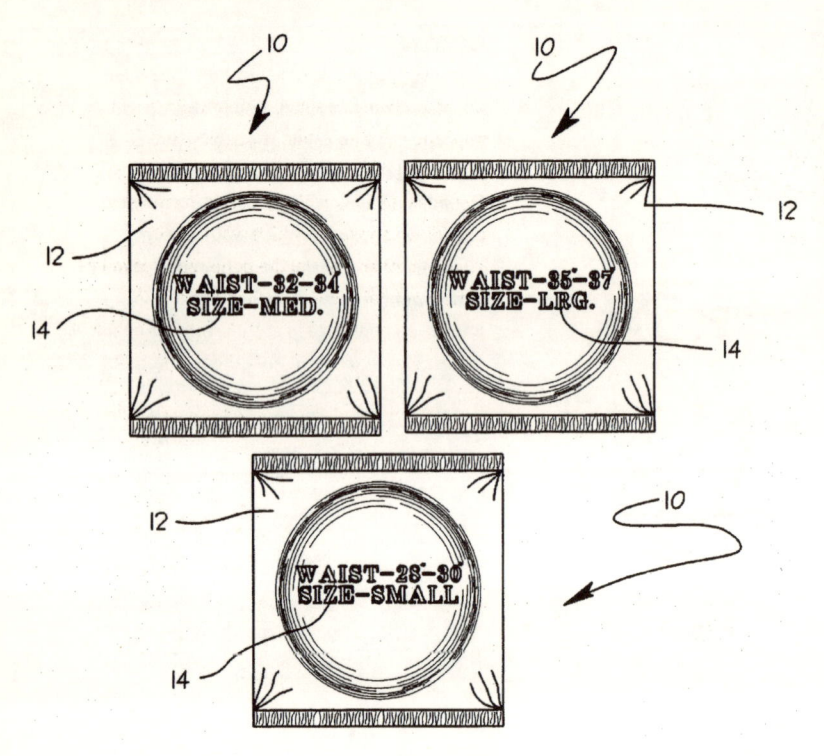

### Abstract

A condom for securely receiving the male sexual organ. The inventive device includes a condom having a cylindrical sheath closed at a distal end and open at a proximal end thereof. Straps extend from the proximal end of the condom and can be positioned about a waist of a male wearer to secure the condom from unintentional removal.

Patent No. 1,511,572
Oct 14, 1924
Jean H. Marshall

# Surgical Appliance

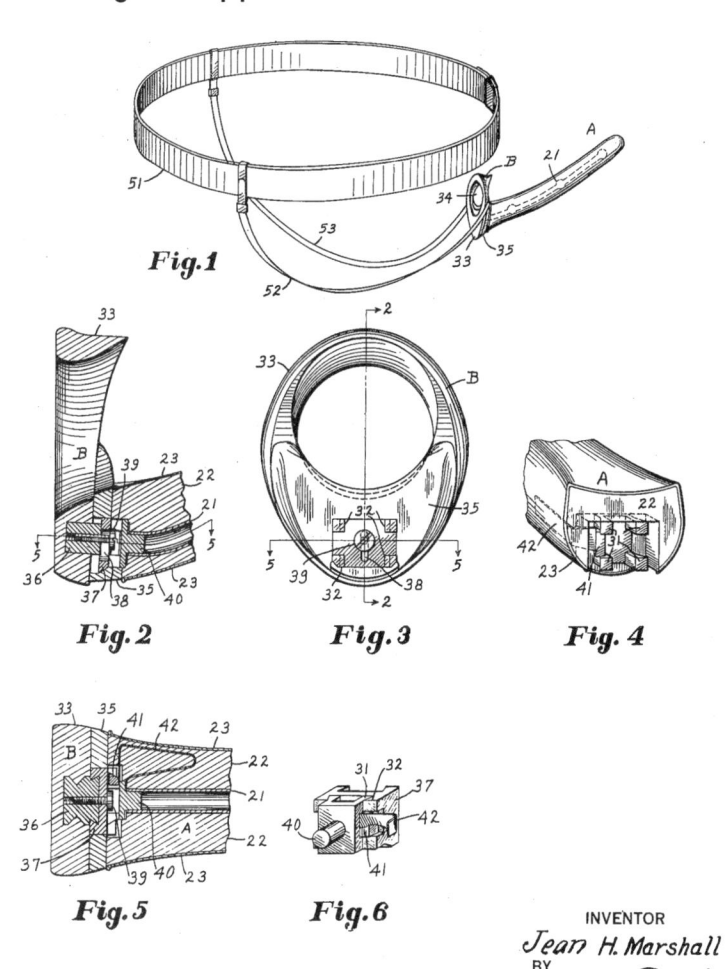

## Abstract

This invention relates to surgical appliances, and is particularly suited for embodiment in appliances for assisting copulation and promoting the attainment of resultant fecundation. It is an object of this invention to provide an appliance which will suitably supplement and assist the penetrative power of a male genital organ. Another object is to provide an appliance of such form as to enable it to suitably supplement the caliber of such an organ during copulation.

Patent No. 5,971,480
Oct 26, 1999
Michael Maschke

## Swinging and/or Spinning, Hanging Seat for Erotic Purposes

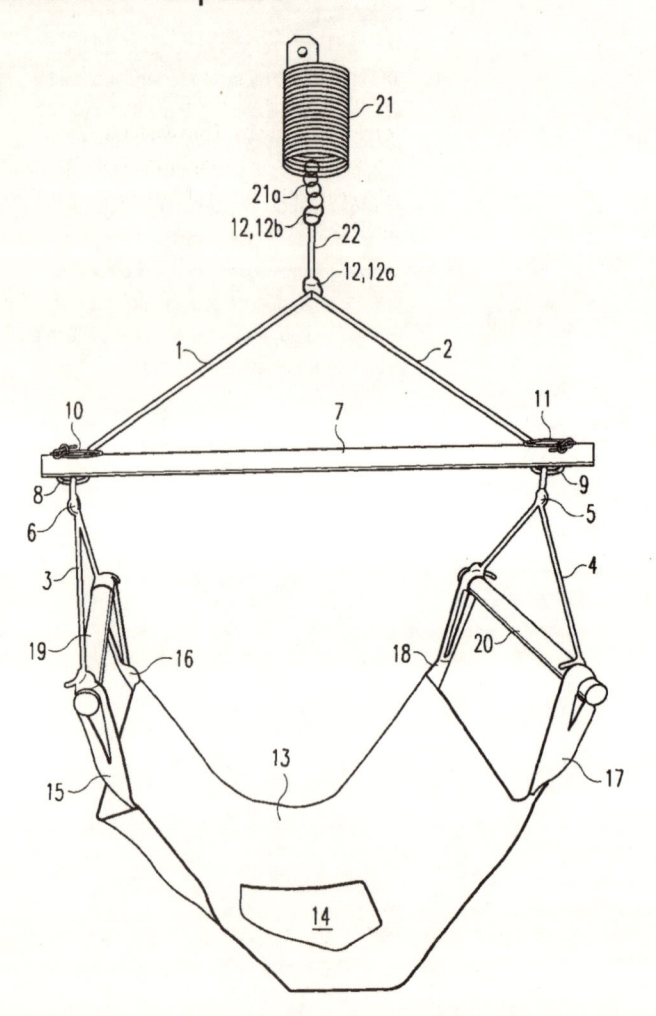

### Abstract

There is disclosed a rotatable seat which comprises a substantially rectangular seat element made of a flexible material and having a centrally disposed hole. The seat element is suspended from two parallel poles which in turn are suspended from the ends of a third pole. The third pole itself is suspended by means of ropes from a fixed point.

Patent No. 4,488,541
Dec 18, 1984
Juan A. S. Garcia

# Therapeutic Adapter

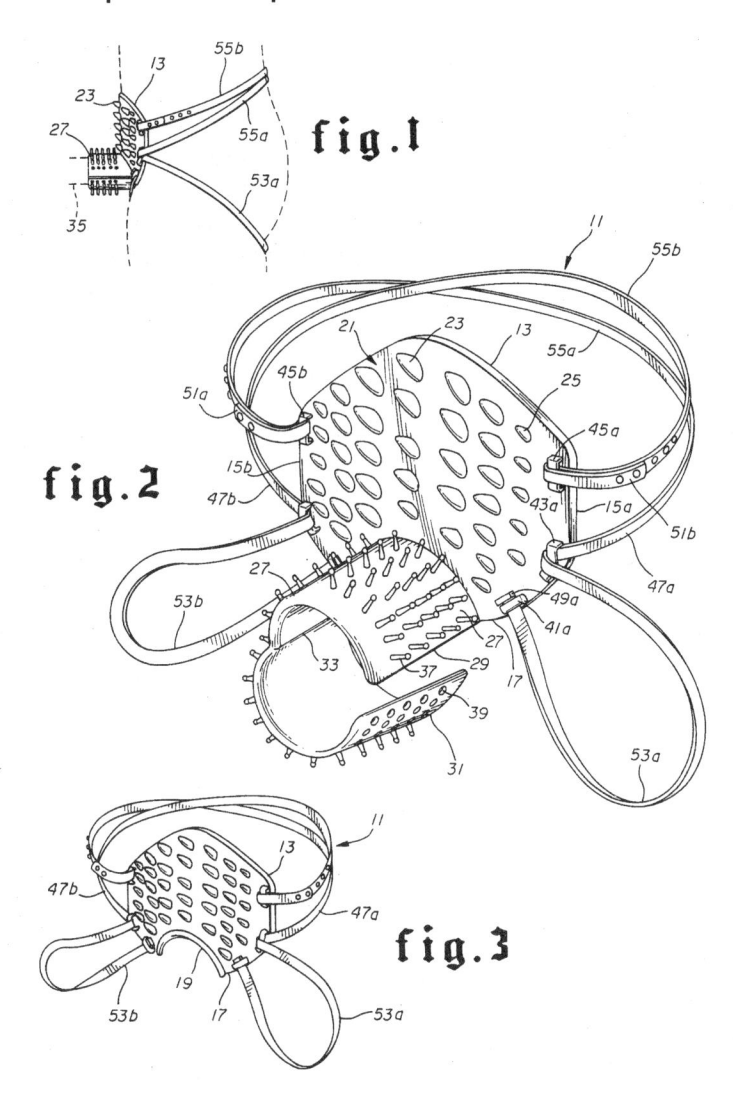

## Abstract

Disclosed is a therapeutic sex aid adapter. The adapter includes a flexible pubic shield having a plurality of monolithically formed inverted conical projections. The adapter may also include a monolithically formed tubular portion. The adapter is held in place by a system of waist and leg belts.

# Therapeutic Aid Apparatus and Method

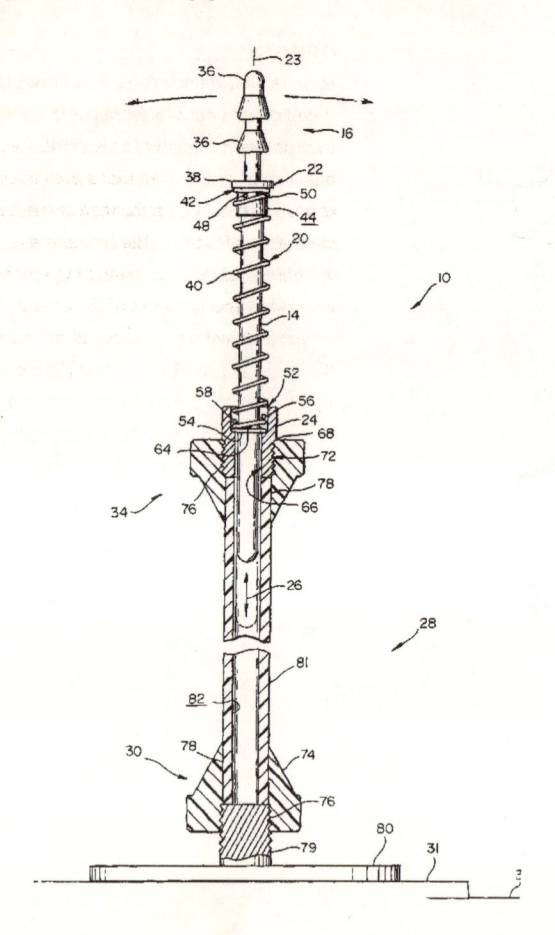

Patent No. US 6,579,228 B2
June 17, 2003
Gary W. Lien

## Abstract

A therapeutic aid includes an elongate centrally disposed shaft with a head coupled to one end thereof for removably receiving a phallus device. To support the shaft in a first extended position, a biasing element is disposed adjacent to the shaft. A retaining member is disposed adjacent to the head for retaining a portion of the biasing element in relation to the shaft. A slide seat is slidingly received by the shaft, and is fixed to an opposing portion of the biasing element such that the shaft is movable from a first extended position where the head is disposed at its furthest point from the slide seat, to a second compressed position where the head is urged toward the slide seat as the slide seat slides along the shaft to compress the biasing element between the retaining member and the slide seat.

Patent No. 3,035,571
May 22, 1962
William R. Jones

# Therapeutic Brassiere

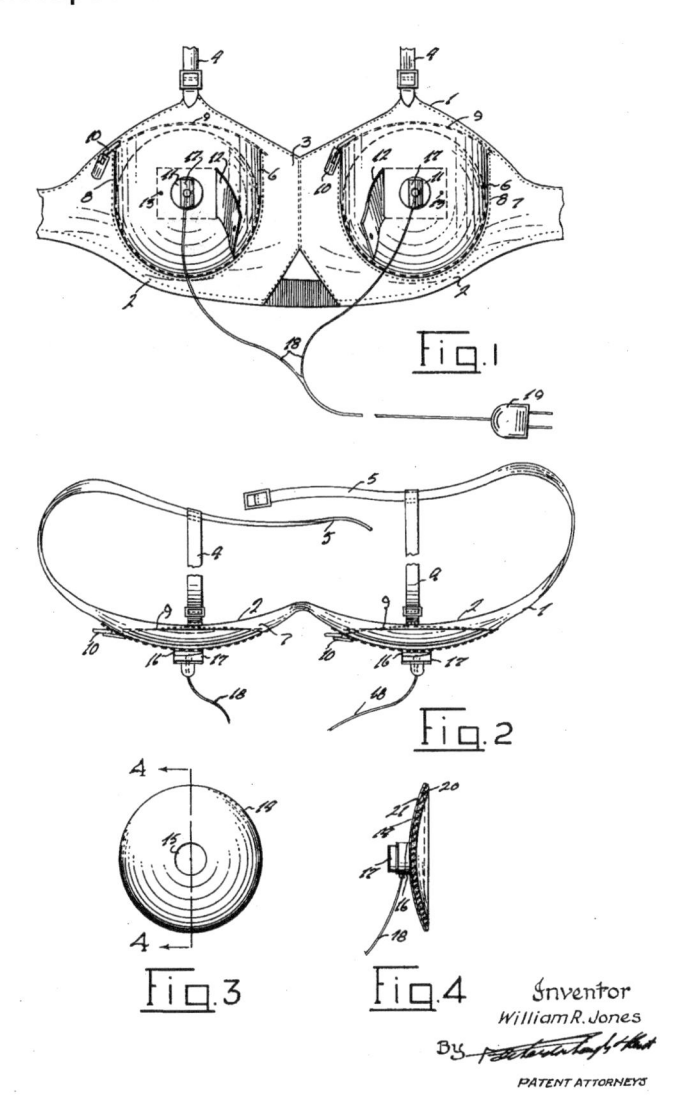

## Abstract

My invention relates to new and useful improvements to brassieres by the incorporation therein of an electrically operated dilator. It is well known that a bust appearance of a woman may be enhanced by increasing the circulation of blood in the breast areas, said increase in circulation promoting enlargement or dilation and firmness of the breast. The principal object and essence of my invention is, therefore, to provide electrical vibrator devices which increase the circulation of blood in the breast areas and promote enlargement or dilation and firmness of the breast.

Patent No. US 6,251,066 B1
June 26, 2001
Juergen Pack

# Thrusting Rod

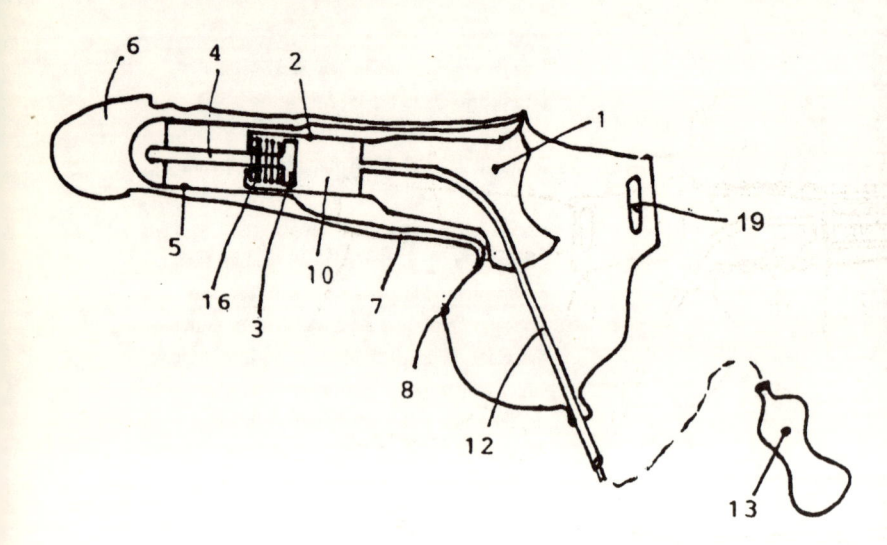

## Abstract

An artificial penis has a cylinder having a cylinder wall enclosing a hollow, a front wall with a first opening and a rear wall with a second opening. A piston rod is guided within the hollow. The piston rod has an initial position in which a first cylinder space is at a maximum and a second cylinder space is at a minimum and an extended position in which the first cylinder space is at a minimum and the second cylinder space at a maximum. A pump supplies a fluid under pressure to move the piston rod in an extending direction. An enclosure having an outer shape of a penis encloses the cylinder and the end of the piston rod. The enclosure has an initial position when the pump is released and an extended position when the pump is actuated.

Fig. 1

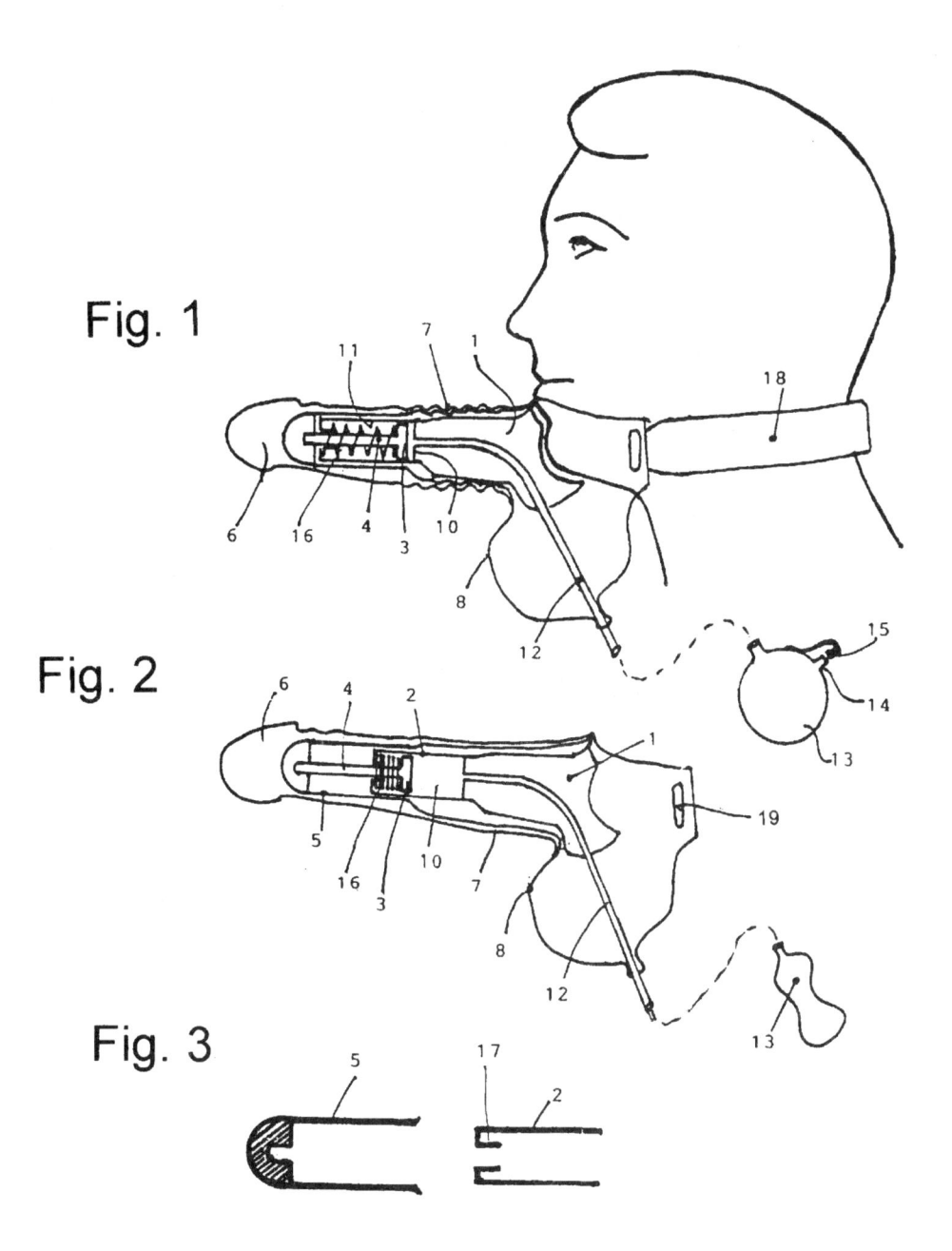

Fig. 2

Fig. 3

Patent No. US 6,179,774 B1
Jan 30, 2001
Jean-Paul Landry

# Vacuum Driven Stimulative Sexual Aid

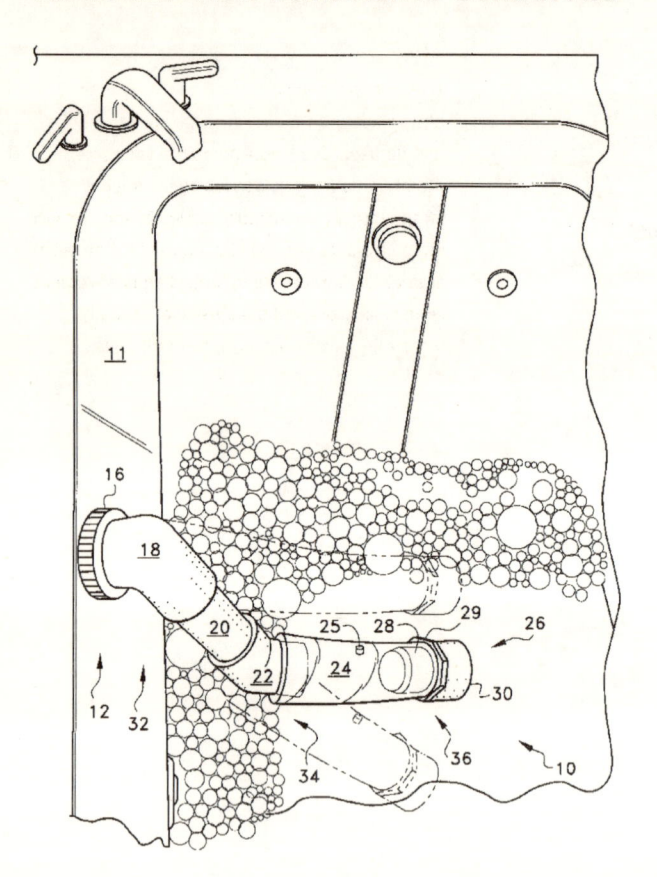

### Abstract

A sexual aid comprises a plurality of interlocking tubes that channel water from a hot tub to the inlet jet, creating a vacuum for inducing blood flow into the erectile tissues of the penis while also producing a pleasurable sensation that massages these tissues. Upon inserting his flaccid penis into the end of the device farthest from the inlet jet and activating the jet mechanism of the tub, a male creates a vacuum that sucks water from the tub through the channel defined by the connected components. The force of the vacuum urges blood into the erectile tissues of the user's penis, ultimately inducing an erection. The influx of water generated by the inlet jet vacuum also massages the penis, contributing to the formation of an erection and creating a pleasurable sensation for the user. The flexible and collapsible properties of tube enable it to better simulate internal female genitalia, further enhancing the sensation that the user experiences.

Patent No. 4,967,767
Nov 6, 1990
Robert L. Harris; Johnnie Carter

# Vaginal Shield for Preventing Sexually Transmitted Diseases

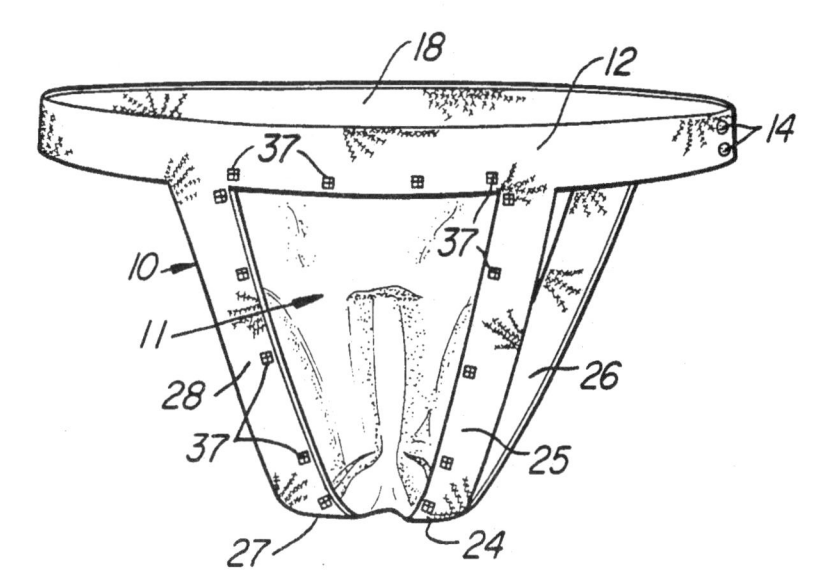

## Abstract

A shield appliance including a shield support strap structure that fits over the lower end of a female user, and a non-porous, elastic shield member, detachably carried by the support strap member, detachably carried by the support strap structure, and positioned over the perineal area of the female use to protect against vaginal contact, and prevent the spread of sexually transmitted diseases, during cunnilingus.

Patent No. 5,377,692
Jan 3, 1995
William Pfeil

# Vibrating Condom

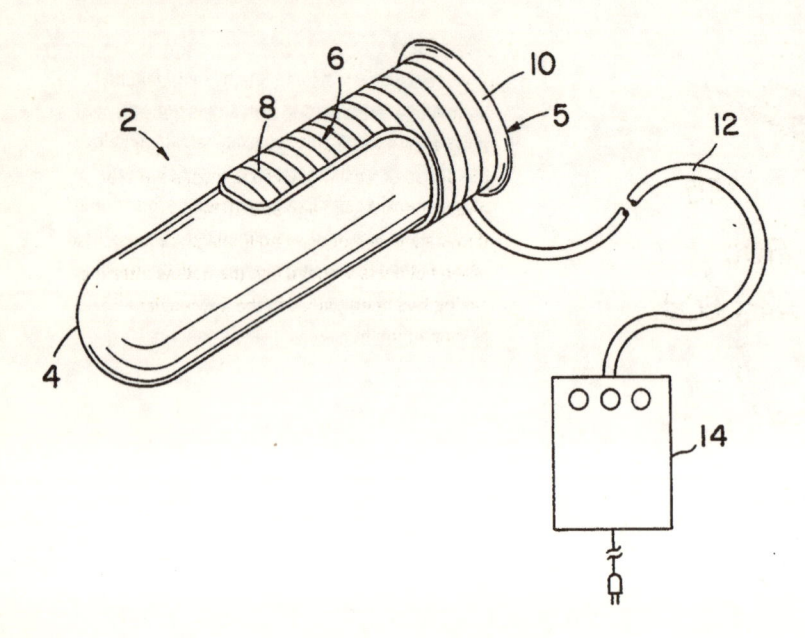

### Abstract

A vibrating condom or device having an inflatable vibrating region or a self-activated vibrating region which contacts the clitoris or vaginal walls. The inflation of such vibrating region is achieved by the transport of air or fluid from a power unit while the self-activated vibrating region could be achieved by an external or imbedded power source.

Patent No. 5,573,499
Nov 12, 1996
Ron McAllister

# Vibrator System

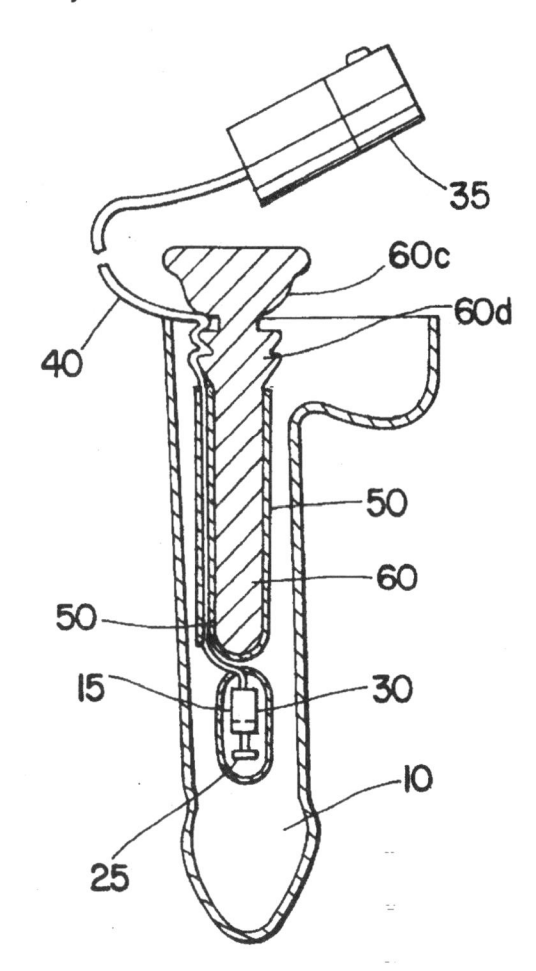

## Abstract

A vibrating device having a body with a hollow including a shaft portion and an impression portion within the hollow which corresponds to the shape of a casing which encloses a motor and spinner. A plug and sheath having dimensions corresponding to the shaft portion of the hollow is wedged into the hollow after the casing has been placed in the impression portion of the hollow.